DENTAL HYGIENE:
The Detection and Removal of Calculus

Anna Matsuishi Pattison, M.S., R.D.H.

Assistant Professor
University of Southern California, NOSANG

Formerly Associate Director,
Dental Auxiliary Occupations
Allied Health Professions Project
Division of Vocation Education
University of California, Los Angeles

and

Jacquelyn Behrens, B.S., R.D.H.

University of Southern California

Formerly Dental Auxiliary Occupations
Allied Health Professions Project
Division of Vocational Education
University of California, Los Angeles

Reston Publishing Company, Inc. *A Prentice-Hall Company*

Reston, Virginia

© 1973 by
RESTON PUBLISHING COMPANY, INC.
A Prentice-Hall Company
Box 547
Reston, Virginia 22090

10 9 8 7 6 5

ISBN: 0-87909-185-1

Library of Congress Catalog Card Number: 72-96758
Printed in the United States of America.

DENTAL HYGIENE:
The Detection and
Removal of Calculus

Occupational Code Designations for the Dental Hygienist

U.S. Office of Education: OE 06.0301; 07.0102
Dictionary of Occupational Titles: DOT 078.368-014

This publication was prepared pursuant to Grant No. 8-0627, Office of Education, U.S. Department of Health, Education, and Welfare. Points of view or opinions were developed on the basis of advisory committee suggestions, survey data, and other sources. They do not, therefore, necessarily represent official Office of Education position or policy.

Foreword

The Division of Vocational Education, University of California, is an administrative unit of the University which is concerned with responsibilities for research, teacher education, and public service in the broad area of vocational and technical education. During 1968 the Division entered into an agreement with the U.S. Office of Education to prepare curricula and instructional materials for a variety of allied health occupations. For the most part, such materials are related to pre-service and in-service instruction for programs ranging from on-the-job training through those on the Associate degree level.

A National Advisory Committee, drawn from government, education, professional associations in the health care field and the lay public, provides guidance and help to the over-all activities of the Allied Health Professions

Project. The following individuals and institutions participate in the activities of this nationwide interdisciplinary body:

Phillip L. Williams, *Chairman*
Vice President, The Times Mirror Company
Los Angeles, California

Lowell Burkett, Executive Director
American Vocational Association
Washington, D.C.

L. M. Detmer, Director
Bureau of Health Manpower and Education
American Hospital Association, Chicago, Illinois

Dale Garell, M.D.
Children's Hospital
Los Angeles, California

John F. Henning, Executive Secretary-Treasurer
California Federation of Labor
San Francisco, California

Joseph Kadish, Ph.D., Acting Chief
Education Program Development Branch
National Institutes of Health, Washington, D.C.

Bernard F. Kamins
Public Relations Consultant
Beverly Hills, California

Ralph C. Kuhli, Director
Department of Allied Medical Professions and Services
American Medical Association, Chicago, Illinois

Leon Lewis, Chief
Division of Occupational Analysis and Employer Services
Manpower Administration, Department of Labor, Washington, D.C.

Walter J. McNerney, President
Blue Cross Association
Chicago, Illinois

Peter G. Meek, Executive Director
National Health Council
New York, New York

Mark J. Musser, M.D., Chief Medical Director
Department of Medicine and Surgery
Veterans Administration, Washington, D.C.

Leroy Pesch, M.D., Deputy Assistant Secretary for Health Manpower
Department of Health, Education, and Welfare
Washington, D.C.

Helen K. Powers, Education Program Specialist
Health Occupations Education
U.S. Office of Education, Washington, D.C.

William M. Samuels, Executive Director
Association of Schools of Allied Health Professions
Washington, D.C.

Dr. William Shannon, Acting Executive Director
American Association of Junior Colleges
Washington, D.C.

Elizabeth Simpson, Ph.D.
Bureau of Research, U.S. Office of Education
Washington, D.C.

John D. Twiname, Commissioner, Social and Rehabilitation Service
Department of Health, Education, and Welfare
Washington, D.C.

C. Gordon Watson, D.D.S., Executive Director
American Dental Association
Chicago, Illinois

Richard S. Wilbur, M.D., Assistant Secretary of Defense
Department of Defense
Washington, D.C.

This document presents work to date in the development of curricula and instructional materials for the Dental Hygienist.

Melvin L. Barlow, Director
Division of Vocational Education
University of California

Professor of Education, UCLA

Principal Investigator
Allied Health Professions Project

Preface

The Allied Health Professions Project, a national curriculum research and development program funded by the U.S. Office of Education, initiated operations in August of 1968 as part of the University of California Division of Vocational Education. This program undertook to develop curricula and instructional materials of a unique and innovative nature for use in training a variety of allied health personnel. The materials were created specifically for those allied health functions that can appropriately be taught in educational programs up through the Associate degree level. Some also can be used for in-service and pre-service instruction in connection with those health-related occupations that utilize on-the-job training.

The basic methodology of the Allied Health Professions Project may be summarized as follows. After extensive FIELD AND LIBRARY RESEARCH, the results were filtered through a NATIONAL TECHNICAL ADVISORY COMMITTEE of practitioners and educators to develop a TASK LIST of all identifiable tasks and functions for each occupation. Data about each of the tasks in the list were obtained through a NATIONAL SURVEY of health care personnel. These data were analyzed and published in a TASK ANALYSIS REPORT. From the task analysis was developed the DESIGN OF THE INSTRUCTIONAL MATERIAL. These included the rationale for the overall teaching strategy, specification of teaching objectives, and division of the instructional unit into MODULES OF INSTRUCTION. The Allied Health Professions Project defines a module as a basic, self-contained instructional package. For each module in the unit, a FIRST TEACHING DRAFT was developed and field-tested extensively until all the the teaching objectives were met in the FINAL TEACHING DRAFT. The final phase of the project was the PRODUCTION AND DISTRIBUTION of these materials.

The development of an instructional unit titled "The Detection and Removal of Calculus" was begun in the fall of 1970, after a survey regarding priority tasks was made of members of the National Technical Advisory Committee for the Dental Auxiliary Occupations and the ADHA Committee on Dental Hygiene Education. This unit of individualized instructional materials is designed to teach dental hygiene students to use the various instruments and aids designed to detect and remove calculus. The five modules in this unit are:

Module I: Fundamental skills for Instrumentation (grasp, finger rest, insertion, angulation, and stroke)

Module II: The Detection of Calculus and Periodontal Pockets (use of the mirror, explorer, periodontal probe, compressed air, and radiographs)

Module III: The Removal of Light to Moderate Calculus (use of the curette, straight sickle, and modified sickle)

Module IV: The Removal of Heavy Calculus (use of the hoe, file, and ultrasonic scaling devices)

Module V: Root Planing Procedure (use of the curette for root planing)

The instructional materials have been spiral-bound in soft covers so that they can easily be used by the students in their intended environment, the dental hygiene laboratory or clinic. Modules I, II, and III are suitable for first-year students and Modules IV and V are designed for second-year students. Although the unit falls naturally into two parts, it would be conceivable and desirable for a progressive student or school to utilize all five modules during the first year. This is feasible because the modular approach allows each student to work and learn at her own rate.

Each module begins with a general introduction, lists of prerequisites and performance objectives, and directions for use of the module. This is followed by a series of skills lessons, each with its own review questions and performance checklists. An answer key and reading assignments for review or enrichment complete the module. Since all important concepts related to each particular skill are included in the module, the need for a lecture before the laboratory or clinic period is virtually eliminated. The student spends most of the period working and learning independently, and the performance checks insure that each student has mastered all necessary skills before moving on to more complex procedures.

The modules were field-tested during the fall of 1971 in six schools of dental hygiene. A limited number of modules also were sent to a select group of dental hygiene educators throughout the country for review and evaluation. Final revision of the modules was completed during the spring of 1973, immediately prior to publication.

Perhaps it should be specified that the procedures described and the nomenclature employed are those typically found in the western part of the United States. It is acknowledged that regional differences will be encountered. There is no intention, therefore, of presenting either procedures or terminology as the only correct approaches or the uniquely authentic nomenclature utilized in the practice of dental hygiene. Individual instructors and practitioners may wish to modify details of this text in line with their own preferences and concepts. It is hoped that the basic material presented will lend itself to such modification without distortion of the initial intent.

A. M. P.
J. B.

Acknowledgements

We are deeply grateful to the many individuals who have given invaluable assistance in the development and preparation of these instructional modules. We would like to thank Mrs. Susan Orloff for her fine work as a contributing writer. Many members of the AHPP Staff assisted in various aspects of the developmental phase. The Project administrators, Dr. Thomas Freeland, Dr. Katherine Goldsmith, and Dr. Miles Anderson have provided excellent counsel and assistance. The constructive criticism and expertise in Instructional Technology which Dr. David Ainsworth contributed to this endeavor are most gratefully recognized. Mrs. Seba Kolb, staff editor, is acknowledged for the many hours of work she devoted to refinement of this material. Miss Charilyn Johnston and Mrs. Elaine Sturdivant are commended for their secretarial skills and patience in typing numerous revisions. We also want to thank Mr. Robert Orr for helping with the final layout of the manuscript.

Several people at neighboring institutions have helped to make this project a combined effort for an educational cause. Mr. Aaron Todd of the Department of Instructional Technology, University of Southern California School of Dentistry, made production of the photographs possible. Special thanks are due Mr. Daniel Wagner, dental photographer, who took the exceptional photographs for the text. Mrs. Ruth Ragland and Mrs. Karoline Waldman of the Department of Dental Hygiene at the University of Southern California made many helpful suggestions and gave generously of their time in consultation. Mrs. Joy Ward and Miss Rosemarie Valentine, Los Angeles City College Department of Dental Hygiene, are also to be thanked for their interest and constructive advice.

We are indebted to Mr. Jim Beauchamp of the Den-tal-ez Manufacturing Company for lending us the dental mannequins which appear in the photographs. This unique and exciting teaching aid, which is designed with transparent gingiva, was indispensible for the preparation of our photographs and it permits a tactile skill to become more visual for the beginning student. Mr. Jack Blatt of the Star Dental Manufacturing Company provided many complimentary instruments, encouragement and an interest in dental hygiene education rarely exhibited by a commercial concern.

The National Technical Advisory Committee for Dental Auxiliary Occupations deserves an expression of gratitude for its early deliberations, which resulted in the establishment of task analyses, and for its continuing interest and advice. A complete roster of the Committee membership is shown on the following pages.

Mrs. Joy Ward (Dental Hygienist)
Director of Dental Hygiene Education
Los Angeles City College
Los Angeles, California

Thomas W. Beckham, Director of Education
American Dental Association
Chicago, Illinois

Dr. Nathan H. Boortz, Chairman
Dental Auxiliary Curriculum Planning Committee
California Community Colleges
Director, Technical Information
Foothill Junior College District
Los Altos Hills, California

Robert M. Gertz
Acting Executive Director
Association of Schools of Allied Health Professions
Washington, D.C.

Harold Globe, D.C.T.
Globe Dental Laboratory
Beverly Hills, California

Otto Kramer, Owner and Operator
Kramer Dental Studios
Minneapolis, Minnesota

Miss Lois K. Kryger
Dental Assistiang Consultant
Division of Dental Health
National Institutes of Health
Bethesda, Maryland

Robert R. Montgomery, D.D.S.
Coordinator, Dental Assistants Program
Oakland Community College, Highland Campus
Union Lake, Michigan

Wayne L. Pack, D.D.S. (Practicing Dentist)
Committee on Dental Health Auxiliary Education
Ogden, Utah

Miss Margaret Ryan
Director, Division of Education
American Dental Hygienist Association
Chicago, Illinois

Charles Strother, D.D.S. (Practicing Dentist)
Chairman, Council on Dental Education
Southern California Dental Association
Glendale, California

Mrs. Hazel Torres
Coordinator of Dental Assisting
College of Marin
Kentfield, California

Miss Rosemarie Valentine
(Dental Hygienist)
Los Angeles, California

William R. Woodworth
Dental Laboratory Training Program
Los Angeles City College
Los Angeles, California

Mrs. Lucille Giles
(Dental Assistant)
Ogden, Utah

Dental Hygiene Subcommittee

Dr. Wayne Pack — *Chairman*
Miss Joy Bebbling
Dr. Nathan Boortz
Miss Margaret Ryan
Miss Rosemarie Valentine

A number of specialists gave valuable assistance. We wish to thank them most sincerely for their conscientious efforts.

Miss Lorna Bonnet
(Dental Hygienist)
Pocatello, Idaho

Mrs. Joan Bradlin
Department of Dental Hygiene
Pasadena City College
Pasadena, California

Miss Kathleen N. Ellegood
Division of Educational Services
American Dental Hygienists Association
Chicago, Illinois 60611

Mrs. Martha H. Fales
University of Washington
School of Dentistry
Department of Dental Hygiene
Seattle, Washington

Mrs. Patricia McLean
School of Dental and Oral Surgery
New York, New York

Dr. Dale Podshadley
Department of Health, Education, and Welfare
Education Research Branch
Division of Dental Health
Bethesda, Maryland

Mrs. Jean Poupard
University of California
School of Dentistry
San Francisco Medical Center
San Francisco, California

Miss Dixie Scoles
Dental Auxiliary Teacher Education
University of North Carolina
Chapel Hill, North Carolina

Mrs. Patricia Wagner
(Dental Hygienist)
Belmont, California

Finally, Mrs. Pattison would like to express special appreciation to Dr. Gordon Pattison, for the many long nights he spent assisting her as a contributing writer, technical editor, proofreader, typist, confidant, cherished companion and friend who settled for peanut butter sandwiches and preserved her sanity throughout the hectic year of writing.

Anna Matsuishi Pattison
Jacquelyn Behrens

Contents

MODULE I

Fundamental Skills for Instrumentation

1. PREREQUISITES

Before beginning work on this module, you must have knowledge of the following subjects, all of which are directly related to the proper use of instruments:

A. PATIENT AND OPERATOR POSITIONING

    (1) posture and body alignment

    (2) positioning the patient

    (3) positioning the operator

B. ORAL ANATOMY

    (1) terminology

    (2) normal oral landmarks

    (3) structure of the gingiva

1

C. DENTAL ANATOMY NOMENCLATURE

D. INTRODUCTION TO THE ORAL PROPHYLAXIS

    (1) role of the dental hygienist

    (2) rationale for oral prophylaxis

The exercises and review questions in this module require this background knowledge. Unless you comprehend the material well, you will encounter difficulty in understanding instructions and performing the skills throughout the module.

    If some review is needed in any of these areas, turn to page 74 and read the suggested assignment for the particular subject. If you are then confident of your knowledge, proceed with the module.

2. PERFORMANCE OBJECTIVES

Performance objectives tell the student, the instructor, and any other interested parties exactly what the student is expected to learn and be able to do upon completion of any course of instruction. Therefore, this module will teach the student to perform only the skills listed in the objectives below, and only these skills will be evaluated on performance tests.

A. GENERAL OBJECTIVE

    Given a mirror, explorer, curette, several extracted teeth with subgingival calculus, and a manikin with artificial subgingival and supragingival calculus, the student will be able to demonstrate the fundamental instrumentation skills that are necessary for the detection and removal of calculus.

B. SPECIFIC OBJECTIVES

    Without the aid of source materials, the student will be able to:

    (1) identify the mirror and explorer, and name the three basic parts of these instruments.

    (2) hold the mirror in the left hand with a modified pen grasp and demonstrate ability to control the instrument by rolling the handle clockwise and counterclockwise between the fingers, smoothly and without slipping.

    (3) hold the explorer in the right hand with a modified pen grasp and demonstrate ability to control the instrument by rolling the handle clockwise between the fingers, smoothly and without slipping.

(4) establish an intraoral finger rest on the occlusal surfaces of the mandibular right bicuspid teeth of the manikin or fellow-student patient.

(5) simulate proper insertion of the explorer on an extracted molar with a short, oblique stroke, keeping the tip flush against the tooth surface.

(6) insert the explorer subgingivally on the buccal surface of the mandibular right first molar of the manikin or fellow-student patient with a short, oblique stroke, keeping the tip flush against the tooth surface.

(7) demonstrate proper adaptation of the explorer to the buccal surface of an extracted molar and the mandibular right first molar of the manikin or fellow-student patient.

(8) name and locate the surfaces and cutting edges of the curette blade.

(9) determine the correct working end of the curette for use:

    (a) in a mesial direction on the buccal surface of the mandibular right first molar of the manikin or fellow-student patient.
    (b) on any other area designated by the instructor.

(10) simulate proper insertion of the curette on an extracted molar with a short, oblique stroke, keeping the face of the blade flush against the tooth surface.

(11) insert the curette subgingivally on the buccal surface of the mandibular right first molar of the manikin or fellow-student patient with a short, oblique stroke, keeping the face of the blade flush against the tooth.

(12) demonstrate working angulation of the curette blade on an extracted molar and on the buccal surface of the mandibular right first molar of the manikin.

(13) demonstrate exploratory strokes with the explorer and curette on an extracted molar, and also on the mandibular right first molar, second bicuspid, and first bicuspid of a manikin with artificial calculus. After completing these exploratory strokes, the student should be able to:

    (a) describe the feeling of subgingival calculus on extracted teeth while using the explorer.
    (b) describe the feeling of subgingival calculus on extracted teeth while using the curette.
    (c) locate with the explorer all artificial subgingival and supra-gingival calculus on the distal, buccal, and mesial surfaces of these three teeth on the manikin.
    (d) locate with the curette all artificial subgingival and supragingival calculus on only the buccal and mesial surfaces of these three teeth.

(14) demonstrate working strokes with the curette on an extracted molar, and also on the mandibular right first molar, second biscuspid, and

first bicuspid of the manikin. After completing these working strokes, the student should be able to:

(a) remove all subgingival calculus from the extracted molar.

(b) remove all artificial subgingival and supragingival calculus from the buccal and mesial surfaces of these three teeth on the manikin.

3. DIRECTIONS FOR USE OF THE MODULE

The following materials and equipment are required for the successful completion of this module:

A pencil
A dental mirror
An explorer
A curette
* Several extracted molars mounted in stone: one without calculus, three or more with calculus on the root surfaces
* A dental manikin with randomly applied artificial calculus

The manikin should be set up at the lab station and adjusted according to directions from your instructor. All other materials and equipment should be laid out on the desk next to the module.

At the end of each Skills Lesson in this module, you will answer review questions pertaining to the particular skill that has just been described. When you are able to answer all questions correctly and perform the skill, ask your instructor for evaluation. If your performance is satisfactory, the instructor will indicate so on the Performance Checklist, and you may then proceed to the next Skills Lesson.

It must be emphasized that, despite all efforts, no textbook, illustration, audiovisual aid, or other instructional material has been proved totally self-sufficient in the field of dental hygiene. The degree of skill necessary to provide quality dental care cannot be attained without the guidance and critical observation of qualified, concerned instructors.

The modules in this unit provide individualized instruction and can be most effectively utilized when each one serves as a "cookbook." As gourmet chefs work in the kitchen, following recipes which include specific ingredients and instructions, the dental hygiene student should work with these modules in the laboratory or clinic following detailed procedural "recipes," which include important concepts and key steps. Leaving out an ingredient in a recipe or measuring it inaccurately may result in a

* This item will be issued by the instructor.

culinary disaster. In this unit, failure to complete any exercise, reading assignment, or test will result in less than quality care for patients in the clinic.

Excellent comprehension of all concepts and skills in a module is imperative, because each module builds upon the previous one. In order to derive the full benefit from this type of instruction, it is of utmost importance that you carefully follow each set of instructions.

4. SKILLS LESSONS

Lesson A: *General Characteristics of Dental Hygiene Instruments*

All dental hygiene instruments consist of three basic parts: the *handle,* the *shank,* and the *working end.* The scaling instrument shown below illustrates the parts of a typical instrument.

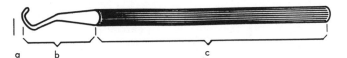

Handle.   Instrument handles may vary in size and may have slight modifications in shape and surface texture to facilitate grasp. The diameter of the handle should be wide enough to allow a comfortable grasp without cramping the fingers or the muscles of the hand. A handle that is too thin is difficult to grasp firmly and therefore inhibits precise control of the instrument. Hollow handles conduct vibrations with greater accuracy and amplification than solid handles. This feature insures good tactile sensitivity during the detection and removal of calculus. The surface texture of the handle may be smooth, ribbed, or scored. A ribbed or scored "waffle-iron" handle is easier to grasp and control than a smooth handle, especially when the fingers become moistened with blood or saliva.

Shank.   The shank of an instrument is thinner than the handle and joins the working end of the instrument to the handle. It is important to consider both the *length* and *angle* of the shank when selecting an instrument. The proper length of the shank for instrumentation is determined by the length of the clinical crown, the depth of the sulcus or pocket, and the area of the mouth to be scaled. An instrument used specifically on anterior teeth where there is no depth or recession will have a short shank, whereas one used in the same area where depth and/or recession exists will demand a longer shank. Also, the angle of the shank may be specifically designed to allow access to particular surfaces of the teeth, such as the mesial or distal surfaces.

Working End.   The working end of the instrument is that part which actually does the work; e.g., the head of a mouth mirror, the tip of an explorer or the blade of a curette. The design of the working end indicates the use of the instrument and determines its classification.

An instrument that has only one working end is called a "single-ended" instrument. There are also "double-ended" instruments, which usually have paired, mirror-image working ends, one on each end of the handle. Working ends may be permanently fixed to the instrument or may be replaceable, cone-socket tips. These tips consist of working ends with threaded shanks, which screw into the handle. Cone-socket tips are economical because only the tip, rather than the entire instrument, need be discarded when the working end becomes worn or broken. It is very important, however, to note that it is not uncommon for these tips to become loosened during scaling.

Instrument Identification.   Instruments are identified by their classification, design name, design number, and manufacturer. The *classification* is determined by the use of the instrument. These classifications include the *periodontal probes, explorers, curettes, sickles, hoes, files,* and *chisels.* Periodontal probes and explorers are detection instruments. The probe is used for measuring the depth of periodontal pockets. The explorer is used to detect calculus, caries, and irregularities in the tooth surface. Curettes are used for gross scaling to remove large calculus deposits, definitive scaling to remove fine calculus, and root planing to smooth and polish the cemental surfaces. Sickles, hoes, files, and chisels are also used in gross calculus removal, but are not suitable for definitive scaling or root planing.

You will be working primarily with the explorer in this module because it is the initial instrument for examination of the mouth and detection of calculus. Later, the curette will be introduced in the skills lesson on angulation. The explorer, the curette, and each of the other types of instruments will be further described in subsequent modules.

In addition to classification, several other factors must be considered for proper identification of an instrument. The instrument *design* bears the name of the school or the individual responsible for its development. Often a *number* provides more specific identification of a design. A double-ended instrument may have a pair of numbers that identify working ends. An instrument of the same design may be manufactured by several different companies. Variations in handle design, type of metal used in fabrication, and blade angulation occur when different companies produce the same instrument. For this reason it is important to be familiar with the *manufacturer's name* as well as the design name.

The Gracey curettes, for example, are produced by several manufacturers. Although the superficial appearance of the instruments may be similar, close examination of the handle, shank, and working end of each will reveal differences that can be very significant when one uses the instrument in the mouth. Gracey is the name of the individual who designed a particular series of curettes, which are numbered from 1 to 14. A Gracey 13-14 curette is an instrument used primarily for removal of calculus from the distal surfaces of posterior teeth. The Gracey 7-8 curette is best suited for buccal, lingual, and mesial surfaces of posterior teeth. In this case, the name of the design alone would not be adequate; the numbers would also have to be specified. Many instruments possess the same numbers, but different designs: the Columbia 13-14 curette is designed for use on the anterior teeth, but is not at all like the Gracey 13-14 curette.

In conclusion, it must be kept in mind that instruments should not be identified by manufacturer alone, design alone, number alone, or classification alone. For effective selection and use of dental hygiene instruments, a thorough knowledge of all four is necessary.

Review Questions for Lesson A: General Characteristics of Instruments

Fill in the correct answer or circle the letter of the best answer.

1. Label the three basic parts of this instrument.

   a. _____ b. _____ c. _____

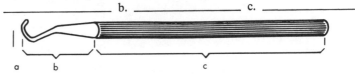

2. Which two characteristics of the shank are determined by the area of the mouth where the instrument should be used?
   a. thickness and length
   b. angle and length
   c. angle and strength
   d. thickness and strength

3. If someone requests a Star Dental Company, Columbia 13-14 curette, you know that:
   a. The classification or type of instrument is _____.
   b. The name of the designer is _____.
   c. The name of the manufacturer is _____.
   d. The design numbers are _____.
   e. The design numbers indicate that this is a _____.
      -ended instrument

MATCH the following instruments with their uses. Write the letter of the *one* phrase which best describes the use of the instrument. Any letter may be used more than once.

_____4. periodontal probe

_____5. explorer

_____6. curette

_____7. sickle

_____8. hoe

_____9. file

a. for use on anterior teeth only
b. for polishing enamel surfaces
c. for gross calculus removal, but not suitable for definite scaling
d. for measuring the depth of periodontal pockets
e. for definitive scaling to remove fine calculus
f. for use on distal surfaces only
g. for detection of calculus and caries

Correct your answers by using the Answer Key on page 72.

Lesson B: *Grasping the Instrument*

The most efficient and stable grasp for all dental hygiene instruments is the *modified pen grasp*. Although other grasps are possible, this slight modification of the conventional or standard pen grasp insures the greatest control in performing intraoral procedures. Now let's see if you can do it!

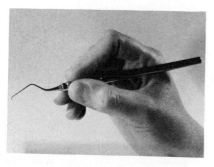

1. Using your right hand, grasp the explorer with the thumb, middle finger, and index finger—as you would a pen. This is the *standard pen grasp*.

2. Now place the pad of the middle finger, instead of the side, against the shank of the instrument. Your thumb and index finger should be opposite to the junction of the handle and the shank.

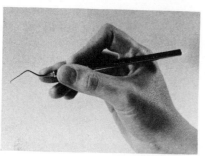

The handle may rest against your hand at any point beyond the first joint of the index finger. This rest point will vary according to the area of instrumentation.

If your hand looks like the one in the second photograph, congratulations! This is the *modified pen grasp*. You have just mastered the first fundamental skill for instrumentation.

Next, try grasping the mouth mirror in your left hand, following the instructions above. Again grasp the explorer in your right hand. During much of the time spent in instrumentation, you will be using the mirror in your left hand for indirect vision; retraction of the lips, cheek, and tongue; or reflection of light while using the explorer or the curette simultaneously in your right hand. Specific instructions on the use of the mirror will be given in the next module.

The *palm grasp* shown in the photograph below is used in manipulation of the air and water syringes, and occasionally for the removal of tenacious deposits. Maneuverability and tactile sensitivity are inhibited considerably by this grasp; however, when used by an experienced operator, it allows the use of great force in dislodging calculus.

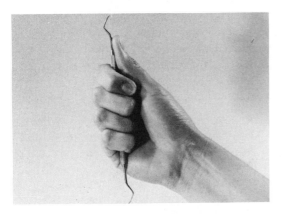

Let's refine your skill with the modified pen grasp by teaching you to rotate these instruments in your fingers. This skill requires accuracy and control, and is essential for the slight, precise manipulations of pointed or sharp instruments in the gingival sulcus. Be sure to grasp your instruments firmly, but not so firmly as to cause blanching of the fingertips. A light grasp will enhance your tactile sensitivity because you will be able to perceive vibrations conducted by the instrument handle. A light grasp will also increase maneuverability of the instrument and cause less muscle fatigue of the hand and fingers.

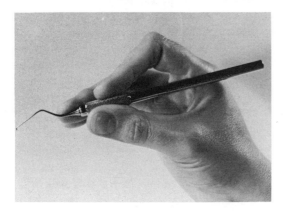

1. Grasp the explorer in your right hand with a *modified pen grasp.*

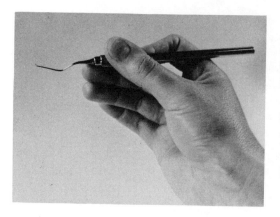

2. *Roll* the instrument very slowly in a clockwise direction by rolling the handle between the thumb, and the opposing index and middle fingers. When you have rolled approximately 180 degrees, roll the handle counterclockwise back to the original position.

Repeat this motion until you can do it very smoothly, without permitting the instrument to wobble.

Try this same exercise with your left hand and rotate the handle of the mirror in the same manner. Can you see why this slight movement of the instrument is so practical and important? The ability to perform this exercise with ease and accuracy means that turning the mirror in the mouth for better indirect vision or adapting the explorer properly around the line angle of a tooth should be duck soup!

Keep this exercise in mind when you begin using strokes with the explorer and the curette. *That slight rolling of the handle is the key to a smooth series of strokes around a tooth.* As you can see in the illustrations below, failure to adapt the instrument to the tooth with this rolling motion will result in laceration of the gingival tissue by the instrument blade or tip and will cause very acute discomfort to the patient. The two sets of drawings show an explorer tip as it is being adapted progressively around the line angle of a root, which is seen in cross section. In both sets, the operator begins with correct adaptation. In the set on the right, the operator has failed to keep the tip closely adapted and the tip has undoubtedly punctured the sulcular epithelium.

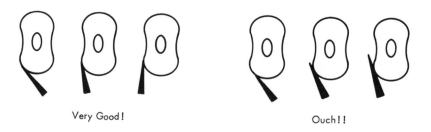

Very Good!   Ouch!!

Review Questions for Lesson B: Grasping the Instrument

Fill in the correct answer or circle the letter of the *one* phrase which best completes the sentence.

1. A very tight grasp will:
   a. increase tactile sensitivity
   b. prevent muscle fatigue of the fingers
   c. increase maneuverability of the instrument
   d. decrease tactile sensitivity

2. Rolling the handle of a sharp instrument between the fingers is important because it:
   a. is a key to adapting the working end around line angles
   b. strengthens the finger muscles
   c. tempers the metal in the handle by friction
   d. can cause laceration of the soft tissue

3. The most efficient, stable grasp for dental hygiene instruments is the _____ grasp.

4. This grasp can be distinguished from the other grasps because:
   a. the thumb, middle finger, and ring finger are used
   b. the pad of the middle finger is placed on the shank
   c. the index finger is placed on the shank
   d. the side of the middle finger is placed against the shank

5. Which drawing shows *incorrect* adaptation of the explorer tip to the surface of the tooth?

a.   b.    c.   d.

6. Incorrect adaptation of the tip as shown above would result in:
   a. gouging of the root surface
   b. failure to detect calculus
   c. laceration of the tissue with the tip
   d. altering the line angle of the tooth

Correct your answers with the Answer Key on page 73.

When you have completed the exercise and answered all of the review questions correctly, ask your instructor to check your performance. If your instructor is occupied and cannot check you immediately, you may go on to the next Skills Lesson while you are waiting.

As you demonstrate the skills listed below, the instructor will evaluate and record your performance. If your ratings are all satisfactory, proceed to the next Skills Lesson. If any of your ratings are unsatisfactory, review the exercise(s) and request another performance check when you are ready.

Performance Checklist for Lesson B: Grasping the Instrument

Name _____

School _____

Date _____

	#1		#2	
	SATISFACTORY	UNSATISFACTORY	SATISFACTORY	UNSATISFACTORY
1. Hold the mirror in the left hand with a modified pen grasp.				
2. Roll the mirror handle clockwise and counterclockwise between the fingers, smoothly and without slipping.				
3. Hold the explorer in the right hand with a modified pen grasp.				
4. Roll the explorer handle clockwise and counterclockwise between the fingers, smoothly and without slipping.				

Instructor _____

Performance Check Time _____

Comments: _____

_____

_____

_____

Lesson C: *Establishing a Finger Rest*

The *finger rest* serves to *stabilize* the hand and the instrument by providing a firm point of rest as movements are made to activate the instrument. A good finger rest *prevents laceration* of the gingiva by poorly controlled instruments and also *insures efficient removal of calculus* because the finger rest acts as a fulcrum when force is applied to dislodge a deposit.

To understand how the finger rest acts as a *fulcrum*, imagine that the instrument is a lever. By resting the pad of your ring finger on a stable surface, such as the teeth, your hand can pivot upon this point and move the instrument in any direction. When the instrument blade encounters a piece of calculus, force is applied to the instrument by rotating the wrist and forearm, and pivoting upon the fulcrum finger. This force enables the instrument blade to remove the deposit from the tooth surface and lift it out of the sulcus. The illustrations below compare the action of a conventional lever and fulcrum with that of a curette and finger rest.

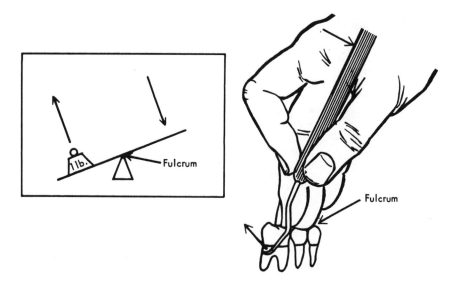

Before learning to establish a finger rest on the manikin, turn to page 71 and perform Exercise A.

A finger rest that is established within the mouth, rather than on the face of the patient, is called an *intraoral finger rest.* An intraoral finger rest that is established as *close to the working area as possible* is preferred. Precise manipulation of the instrument and good leverage for the removal of calculus become more difficult as the finger rest moves further away from the working area. An extraoral finger rest on the lips or face of the patient is possible, but is dangerous because the skin is supple and does not provide a firm point of rest. An inexperienced operator using an extraoral finger rest could easily allow a sharp instrument to slip and injure the patient.

This exercise may be performed on a manikin or a fellow-student patient. If a manikin is preferred, set up the manikin at your laboratory station according to directions from your instructor. Adjust the manikin head and your body according to the principles of good patient and operator positioning. Position the manikin head as if it were a real patient in a dental chair, with the patient at your right side and his mouth at your elbow level.

If a fellow-student patient is chosen, seat the patient and yourself, again according to the principles of positioning. You will need a sterilized mouth mirror and explorer. Before beginning this exercise you will have to refer to Module II, page 75 to learn the mirror finger rest for the lower right posterior-buccal aspect.

You will be establishing a finger rest on the mandibular right bicuspids. The head of the patient should be turned slightly to the left to allow better access and vision.

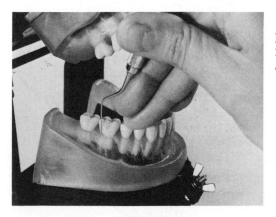

1. Grasp the explorer with a modified pen grasp. Place the pad of your ring finger on the occlusal surfaces of the mandibular right bicuspids.

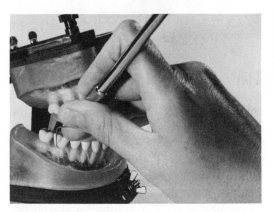

2. If the maxillary arch is limiting movement, rotate your wrist slightly from right to left so your hand is more buccal to the maxillary arch.

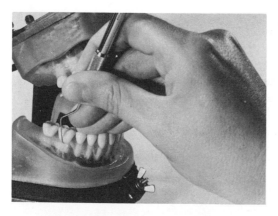

3. Now lift your wrist until the handle is as close to parallel with the long axis of the first molar as possible.

Note: It is impossible to achieve perfect parallelism on the buccal and especially the lingual of posterior teeth. It is more important to remember that, regardless of the handle position, the tip of the explorer must be adapted properly and short, oblique strokes must be used.

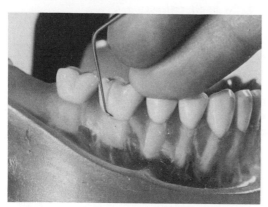

4. Place the explorer tip on the buccal surface of the first molar just above the free margin of the gingiva. Make sure the tip is directed mesially.

Note: The very end of the explorer is called the *point*. The 1 to 2 mm of the working end adjacent to the point is called the *tip*.

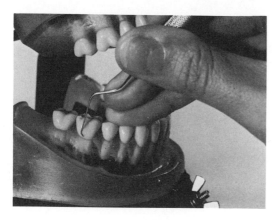

5. Begin the short rocking motion as you did in Exercise A by rotating your wrist from left to right. Keep your wrist and elbow level with your hand or above it.

Limit the movement of the tip to an eighth of an inch up and down so the side of the tip rubs gently against the enamel surface. This movement will be refined later to become a stroke.

You have just learned how to establish an intraoral finger rest. Can you see why a finger rest on the lips, chin, face, or even no finger rest at all, is unstable? To further illustrate this point, try moving the explorer tip up and down on the eighth of an inch from the free margin without any fulcrum at all. Did you feel a little shaky? Just imagine how dangerous a sharp instrument could be with so little control!

Also try moving your finger rest further and further away from your working area. Does your ability to control the instrument diminish as your finger rest moves away? Do you think you could remove a piece of tenacious calculus from the first molar with your finger rest on the incisors?

Review Questions for Lesson C: Establishing a Finger Rest

Fill in the correct answer or circle the letter of the *one* phrase which best completes the sentence.

1. A good finger rest is established by placing the pad of the _____ finger on the teeth.

2. While activating the instrument, the finger rest acts as a:
   a. pivot point for movement
   b. stabilizing point for the hand
   c. fulcrum for the removal of calculus
   d. all of the above

3. The best finger rest for the use of dental hygiene instruments is the:
   a. intraoral rest on the attached gingiva
   b. intraoral rest closest to the working area
   c. extraoral rest on a bony area
   d. intraoral rest with the middle finger

4. Which type of finger rest, extraoral or intraoral, is considered safer? Why?

Correct your answers with the Answer Key on page 73.

Performance Checklist for Lesson C: Establishing a Finger Rest

Name _____

School _____

Date _____

	#1		#2	
	SATISFACTORY	UNSATISFACTORY	SATISFACTORY	UNSATISFACTORY
5. Establish an intraoral finger rest on the occlusal surfaces of the mandibular right bicuspids of the manikin or fellow-student patient.				

Instructor _____

Performance Check Time _____

Comments: _____

_____

_____

_____

Lesson D: *Inserting the Instrument*

Inserting the instrument into the gingival sulcus is the next important step in instrumentation. The instrument must be inserted carefully into the sulcus with a *short, oblique stroke.* This is best accomplished by first positioning the handle of the instrument so that it is as close to parallel with the long axis of the tooth as possible. This will facilitate proper adaptation of the working end to the tooth surface. Now the instrument can be inserted into the sulcus *until the resistance of the epithelial attachment is felt on the back of the working end.* The epithelial attachment is soft, but resilient— somewhat like a taut rubber band. It is important to avoid plunging down into the sulcus with a vertical pushing motion because the sharp instrument tip could easily pierce the attachment and cause acute pain. The working end of the instrument must extend to the depth of the sulcus or pocket to insure thorough calculus detection and removal. Instrumentation that fails to remove calculus from this area is of limited value. Even if all other calculus is removed, one small piece left at the epithelial attachment will continue to harbor bacterial plaque and the periodontal disease process will go on.

Turn to Page 72 and perform Exercises B and C before proceeding further.

Now let's go through the basic steps of insertion on the mounted extracted molar without calculus. This exercise will enable you to see how an instrument should be inserted subgingivally without having your vision obstructed by the gingiva.

INSERTING THE EXPLORER

Exercise on Extracted Tooth

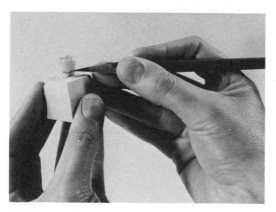

1. Hold the mounted extracted molar with your left hand. Use your pencil to draw a line around the tooth about 3 mm below the cemento-enamel junction (CEJ). This line will represent the epithelial attachment. Imagine that the gingival sulcus extends from the pencil line to just above the CEJ.

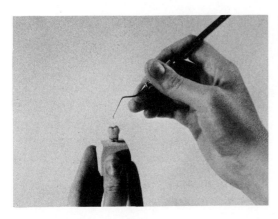

2. Hold the mounted molar by the stone base, as if it were a mandibular molar with the buccal surface toward you. Pick up the explorer with your right hand, using a *modified pen grasp.*

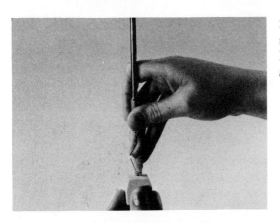

3. Establish a *finger rest* on the occlusal surface of the molar with your ring finger. Make sure that the *handle of the explorer is parallel with the long axis of the tooth.*

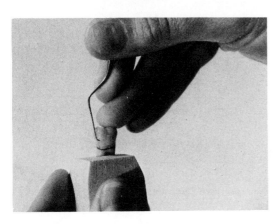

4. Adapt the working end of the explorer to the buccal surface of the molar about 2 mm above the CE junction. Make sure that the *tip is directed mesially* and is lying flat against the tooth at the distal line angle.

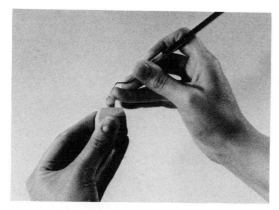

5. Insert the tip by first lowering your wrist and rocking back on your finger rest slightly until the tip is pointing straight down into the sulcus. *Relax your grasp* for ease of insertion.

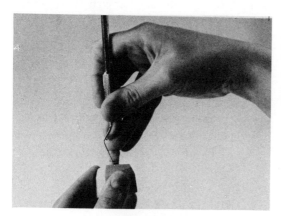

6. Lift your wrist and rock forward until your handle is parallel with the long axis of the tooth again. This *short, oblique stroke* will allow the tip to slide down into the sulcus smoothly without injuring the epithelial attachment.

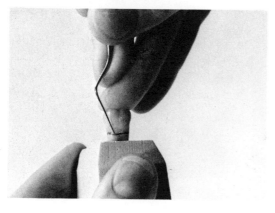

7. If the tip is adapted so that it is flush against the tooth, and the back of the tip is resting on the pencil-line attachment, you've done it!

EXERCISE ON MANIKIN OR PATIENT

Now you will try inserting the explorer on the manikin or fellow-student patient. This time, however, you will have to rely totally on your tactile sensitivity and knowledge of dental anatomy, because the manikin's teeth will be covered with artificial gingiva and the patient's teeth with natural gingiva. Try to visualize exactly what you did when you practiced on the extracted molar, as you work on the manikin's or fellow-student patient's mandibular right first molar in this exercise.

For clarification of the insertion technique: you have just simulated insertion into a 3 mm sulcus on the extracted tooth. If you plan to work on a fellow-student patient, keep in mind that in a healthy mouth, the sulcus may be less than 1 mm in depth. Insertion will be restricted to a smaller area, and greater finesse will be required of your technique.

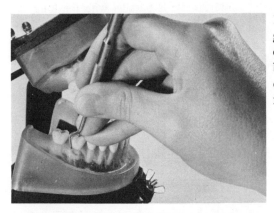

1. Hold the explorer with a modified pen grasp and establish a finger rest on the occlusal surfaces of the mandibular right bicuspids. Position the handle so it is as close to parallel with the long axis of the first molar as possible.

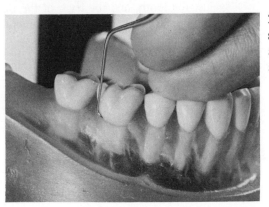

2. Adapt the explorer tip to the buccal surface of the first molar at the distal line angle. The tip should be directed mesially and should be lying flat against the tooth.

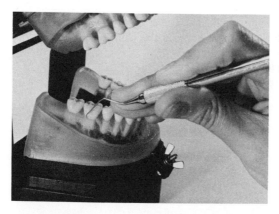

3. Gently insert the tip subgingivally by first lowering the handle and rocking back on your finger rest until the tip is pointing straight down into the sulcus.

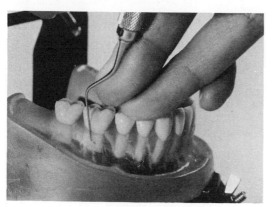

4. Lift your wrist and rock forward until your handle is again parallel with the long axis of the tooth. This motion will activate a *short, oblique stroke.* Try to visualize the tip as it slides down into the sulcus. *Keep as much of the working end as possible in contact with the tooth surface* to insure the greatest degree of tactile sensitivity.

Review Questions for Lesson D: Inserting the Instrument

1. Prior to inserting an instrument, its handle should be positioned so it is as close to _____ with the long axis of the tooth as possible.

2. Calculus at the bottom of the sulcus or pocket cannot be felt or removed unless the instrument is inserted:

    a. to the epithelial attachment
    b. to the cemento-enamel junction
    c. with a plunging vertical stroke
    d. to the distal line angle

3. The instrument should be inserted with a:

    a. short, oblique stroke
    b. vertical pushing motion
    c. short, pulling motion
    d. plunging vertical stroke

4. If the instrument fails to remove calculus at the epithelial attachment, the periodontal disease process will continue because the calculus:
    a. is rough
    b. harbors bacterial plaque
    c. presses against the tissue
    d. decomposes

Correct your answers with the Answer Key on page 73.

Name _____

School _____

Date _____

		#1		#2	
		SATISFACTORY	UNSATISFACTORY	SATISFACTORY	UNSATISFACTORY
6.	Properly adapt the explorer to the buccal surface of an extracted molar.				
7.	Simulate proper insertion of the explorer on an extracted molar with a short, oblique stroke, keeping the tip flush against the tooth.				
8.	Properly adapt the explorer to the buccal surface of the mandibular right first molar of the manikin or fellow-student patient.				
9.	Insert the explorer subgingivally on the buccal surface of the mandibular right first molar of the manikin or fellow-student patient with a short, oblique stroke, keeping the tip flush against the tooth surface.				

Instructor _____

Performance Check Time _____

_____

_____

_____

_____

INSERTING THE CURETTE

You have learned the steps for insertion of an explorer, so let's move on to the curette. Since this is your first exposure to an instrument with cutting edges, there are several important facts related to curette design that you should learn before going further.

Like all other dental hygiene instruments, the curette has a handle, a shank, and a working end. A curette may be single-ended or double-ended. In either case, the working ends of the curettes come in pairs, which are mirror images of each other.

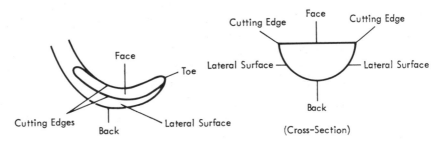

The drawings above show that the curette blade is curved to adapt well to the curvatures of the teeth and that the curette possesses *two cutting edges,* which meet to form a rounded tip or *toe.* Only one cutting edge is actually used against the tooth surface while calculus is being removed. This is why the blade must be positioned carefully to prevent laceration of the soft tissue by the cutting edge that is free or by the edge of the toe.

The sides or *lateral surfaces* of the blade extend from each cutting edge and curve around to merge and form the convex *back* of the blade. The smooth, convex back of the blade allows the cutting edge of the curette to be used in the deepest area of a sulcus or pocket with less possibility of soft tissue damage than with any other scaling instrument. For this reason, *the curette is considered to be the most effective instrument for complete removal of calculus and for smoothing the root surface.*

The flat surface of the blade, which lies between the two cutting edges, is called the *facial surface* or simply the *face* of the blade. The relationship between the face of the blade and the tooth surface is important in insertion and will be discussed later in this module.

You will learn more about curette design and its relationship to function in MODULE III: The Removal of Light to Moderate Calculus, which is devoted entirely to the use of the curette and the sickles. What you have learned now will enable you to move on to solve a basic dilemma that confronts each and every beginning dental hygiene student: How does one determine the correct end of the curette to be used in any given area of the mouth?

Determining the Correct Working End

The working ends of a curette are often paired, enabling you to work on all surfaces of the teeth with a single instrument. A curette of this nature is described as "universal." This name will seem rather ridiculous only until you have learned to use the right end in the right place at the right time. The following guidelines will help you determine this quickly and easily: When the handle of the curette is parallel to the long axis of the tooth, the correct working end of the curette is that blade that curves in the direction in which you wish to scale, and the face of that blade should be close against the tooth so that the face of the blade can only partially be seen. If you can easily see the shiny face of the blade, there is a sharp cutting edge that is free to cause trauma if placed subgingivally. Always remember that there is an opposite cutting edge that is free each time you place the curette against a tooth!

Let's try to find the correct working end of the curette for a few areas on the manikin or fellow-student patient. Concentrate on the design of the blade as you follow instructions. *In this exercise you will be selecting the correct end of the curette for use in a mesial direction on the buccal surface of the mandibular right first molar.*

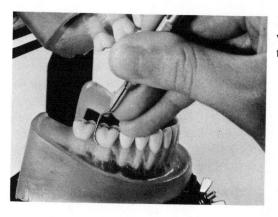

1. Grasp the curette close to the correct working end and establish a finger rest on the mandibular right bicuspids.

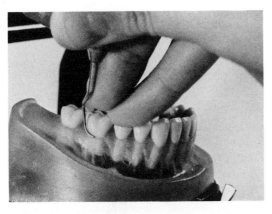

2. Place the curette blade against the buccal surface of the first molar so that it is directed mesially.

Make sure that the handle is as close to parallel with the long axis of the tooth as possible.

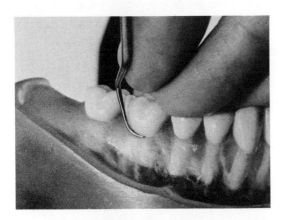

3. The face of the blade should be close against the tooth so it can only be partially seen. This is the CORRECT END of the curette for removal of calculus.

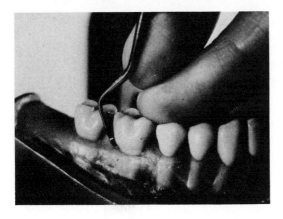

4. If the shiny face of the blade can be seen easily, there is a sharp cutting edge that is free to cause trauma to the soft tissue. Can you see it? Then this is definitely the WRONG END of the curette for removal of calculus.

Review Questions for Lesson D: Inserting the Instrument (cont.)

5. Draw a cross-section of the curette blade and label *each* surface and cutting edge.

6. The curette is called a "universal" instrument because it:
   a. is used by hygienists all over the U.S.
   b. has more than one cutting edge
   c. is most effective in removal of calculus
   d. adapts to all surfaces of the teeth

7. The design feature of the curette blade that allows it to be used in the deepest area of the sulcus or pocket with the least possibility of tissue damage is the:
   a. convex back
   b. opposite cutting edge
   c. face
   d. lateral surfaces

8. Which of the guidelines listed below are essential to determining the correct end of the curette for use on a specific tooth?
   1. handle parallel to the long axis of the tooth
   2. blade curves in direction in which you wish to scale
   3. blade curves away from direction in which you wish to scale
   4. face of blade can only be partially seen
   5. face of blade is easily seen
   6. opposite cutting edge is free

   a. 1,3,4
   b. 1,2,4
   c. 2,4,6
   d. 1,2,5,6

Correct your answers with the Answer Key on page 73.

Performance Checklist for Lesson D: Inserting the Instrument (Cont.)

Name _____

School _____

Date _____

	#1		#2	
	SATISFACTORY	UNSATISFACTORY	SATISFACTORY	UNSATISFACTORY
10. Name and locate the surfaces and cutting edges of the curette blade.				
11. Determine correct working end of curette for use: a. in a mesial direction on the buccal surface of the mandibular right first molar of the manikin or fellow–student patient.				
b. on any other area designated by the instructor.				

Instructor _____

Performance Check Time _____

Comments: _____

_____

_____

_____

INSERTION ON AN EXTRACTED TOOTH

Now that you have determined the correct end of the curette to use on the mandibular right molar, you can learn to insert the curette on that tooth. Inserting the curette is essentially the same as inserting the explorer, but, as you might guess, the difference in the design of the working ends requires some modification of the procedure.

When the explorer is inserted, the *tip* of the instrument is laid flat against the tooth surface. When the curette is inserted, the *face* of the curette blade should be adapted to the tooth surface. This allows smooth insertion of the curette blade and eliminates the danger of lacerating the tissue with a free cutting edge or causing painful distension of the gingival tissue by an open-angled blade. Let's try it on the buccal surface of the extracted molar without calculus.

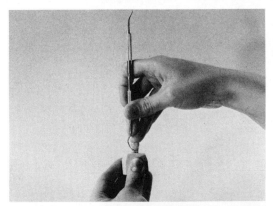

1. Hold the curette with a modified pen grasp and establish your occlusal finger rest. Make sure that you are using the correct end of the curette.

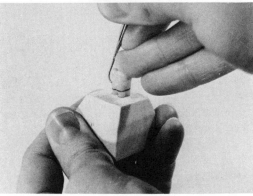

2. Place the face of the curette blade flush against the buccal surface of the tooth at the distal line angle.

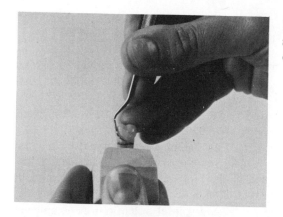

3. Insert the blade with a short, oblique stroke, keeping the face of the blade as close to the tooth as possible.

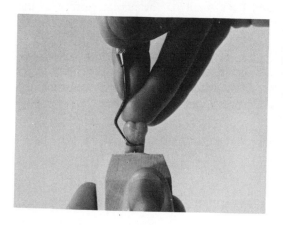

4. When the epithelial attachment is reached, the curved back of the blade should be resting on the attachment, and the face of the blade should be as flush against the tooth as possible.

INSERTION ON MANIKIN OR PATIENT

After you have practiced inserting the curette on the extracted molar, proceed with the exercise on the mandibular right molar of the manikin or fellow-student patient. Follow the same instructions, but remember that the gingiva will prevent you from actually seeing that the blade is flush against the tooth, so you will have to rely on your tactile sense to visualize exactly what your instrument is doing subgingivally.

Now that you have learned to insert these instruments, you are half-way there. You have slipped down to the epithelial attachment gracefully, but how will you come back out of the sulcus with as much ease and agility? With patience, perseverance, and much repetition you will learn this secret of dental hygiene before the day is over!

NOTES AND OBSERVATIONS

Lesson E: *Adapting or Angulating the Instrument*

Adaptation.   The term *adaptation* refers to the act of placing the working end of an instrument against the tooth surface. Although the term is used in reference to many different types of instruments, it is more often used for instruments that do not possess cutting edges, such as the explorer or periodontal probe. These types of instruments should be adapted so that as much of the working end as possible is flush or nearly flush against the tooth. By adapting these instruments close to the surface, distension and injury of the gingival epithelium is prevented and maximum tactile sensitivity is gained.

Angulation.   Any instrument that has cutting edges must be angulated for effective calculus removal. Angulation is also referred to in this context as *tooth-blade relationship.* For this procedure, the face of the blade and the tooth surface should form an angle of more than 45 degrees and less than 90 degrees. If angulation is less than 45 degrees, the cutting edge will not bite into or engage the calculus properly and therefore will slide over the deposit. If angulation is more than 90 degrees, the lateral surface of the blade, rather than the cutting edge, will be against the tooth, and no calculus will be removed.

Also, because the curette has two cutting edges, angulation of 90 degrees or more would mean that the free cutting edge against the sulcular epithelium would lacerate or remove soft tissue. In some instances when the tissue is very swollen and the sulcular epithelium is diseased, the degenerated sulcular lining is deliberately removed with the cutting edge. This advanced procedure is called *soft tissue curettage.*

The illustrations below show the curette blade in cross-section as it is placed against the tooth surface at various angulations.

0 DEGREES	LESS THAN 45	45 DEGREES	MORE THAN 90
Correct angulation for insertion	DEGREES Not open enough for calculus removal	Correct angulation for calculus removal	DEGREES Too wide for calculus removal OUCH!

It is essential that correct angulation and adaptation be maintained at all times to insure optimal detection and complete removal of calculus. As instruments are used on the tooth surface, each line angle, developmental groove, and furcation must be anticipated. The surface of the tooth is by no means static. It is a series of fairly predictable bulges and depressions, which must be pursued by your instruments. Practicing on extracted teeth and the manikin with a keen awareness of dental anatomy will prepare you to adapt and angulate the instruments on a real patient.

You have already mastered proper adaptation of the explorer to the tooth surface during the exercises on insertion. You have also had some experience in angulation of the curette. When? Remember that the blade of the curette was flush against the tooth during insertion? *The proper angulation for insertion of the curette is 0 degrees.* The curette is inserted and held at 0 degrees until the epithelial attachment is reached; then a working angulation of 45 to 90 degrees is established. After working angulation has been established, strokes may be activated for the removal of calculus.

Curette Angulation: Extracted Tooth

Let's try to establish correct working angulation with the curette on the extracted molar without calculus. Be sure to select the correct end of the curette for the buccal surface.

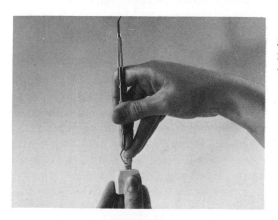

1. Grasp the curette with a modified pen grasp and establish your occlusal finger rest. Your handle should be parallel with the long axis of the tooth.

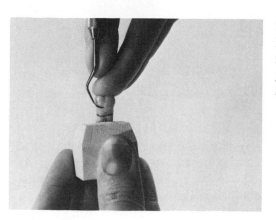

2. Place the curette blade on the distal line angle of the buccal surface about 2 mm above the CEJ. *The blade should be flush against the tooth surface for proper insertion.* Remember, 0 degrees!

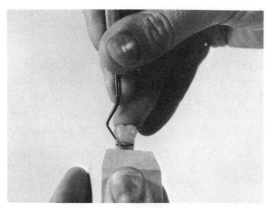

3. Insert the blade to the epithelial attachment with a short, oblique stroke. The curved back of the blade should be against the attachment, and angulation should still be at 0 degrees.

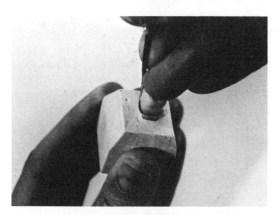

4. Now rotate your wrist and forearm very slightly from right to left, pivoting on your finger rest. This slight movement should be enough to open the angle between the face of the blade and the tooth surface. Open the angle first to 45 degrees.

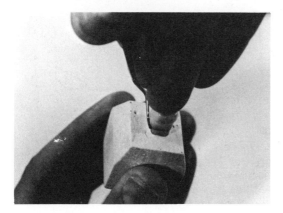

5. Keep the full length of the cutting edge against the tooth and open the angulation slowly to 90 degrees. Open and close the angulation from 0 to 90 degrees several times.

Carefully observe the relationship of the blade and the cutting edges to the tooth surface as you move the blade. Also try to visualize the relationship of the back of the blade and the free cutting edge to the sulcular epithelium.

CURETTE ANGULATION: MANIKIN OR PATIENT

When you have completed this exercise, try to establish working angulation with the curette on the mandibular right molar of the manikin. Insert the curette blade on the buccal surface of the first molar and follow the instructions as you did on the extracted molar. As with insertion, you will have to rely entirely on your tactile sense to determine how to angulate the curette blade.

Review Questions for Lesson E: Adapting or Angulating the Instrument

1. Adapting the face of the curette blade to the tooth allows insertion without:
      a. tissue laceration with the free cutting edge
      b. distension of sulcus by open-angled blade
      c. discomfort of the patient
      d. all of the above

2. Which drawing best illustrates correct angulation of the curette for insertion of the blade?

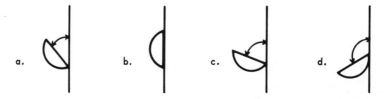

3. Which drawing best illustrates correct angulation of the curette for removal of calculus?

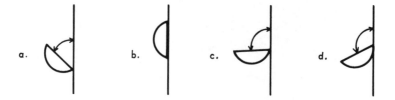

4. The correct angulation of the curette for the removal of calculus is:
      a. more than 40 degrees but less than 15 degrees
      b. less than 90 degrees but more than 45 degrees
      c. more than 90 degrees but less than 45 degrees
      d. less than 100 degrees

Read these statements before answering the next two questions.
   1. The cutting edge would be against the tooth.
   2. The lateral surface would be against the tooth.
   3. Calculus would be removed effectively.
   4. Calculus would not be removed effectively.
   5. The free cutting edge would remove soft tissue.

5. Which of the above statements would apply if angulation of the curette were more than 90 degrees?

    a. 1,3
    b. 1,3,5
    c. 2,4,5
    d. 2,3,5

6. Which of the above statements would apply if angulation of the curette were less than 45 degrees?

    a. 1,3
    b. 1,4
    c. 1,4,5
    d. 2,4

Correct your answers with the Answer Key on page 73.

Performance Checklist for Lesson E: Adapting or Angulating the Instrument

Name _____

School _____

Date _____

		#1		#2	
		SATISFACTORY	UNSATISFACTORY	SATISFACTORY	UNSATISFACTORY
12.	Simulate proper insertion of the curette on an extracted molar with a short oblique stroke keeping the face of the blade flush against the tooth surface.				
13.	Demonstrate working angulation of the curette blade on an extracted molar.				
14.	Insert the curette subgingivally on the buccal surface of the mandibular right first molar of the manikin with a short, oblique stroke keeping the face of the blade flush against the tooth surface.				
15.	Demonstrate working angulation of the curette blade on the buccal surface of the mandibular right first molar of the manikin.				

Instructor _____

Performance Check Time _____

Comments: _____

_____

_____

_____

Lesson F: *Activating a Stroke*

An instrument may be activated by either a pushing or a pulling force. The pulling force is usually preferred for the two general types of strokes: the *exploratory stroke* and the *working stroke*. Both of these are used constantly and interchangeably during instrumentation.

Exploratory Stroke. The exploratory stroke is a light "feeling" stroke, which is used primarily with explorers to detect calculus, but is also used with scaling instruments to search out deposits. The instrument *handle is grasped lightly* to allow maximum tactile sensitivity, and the tip or blade is drawn from the epithelial attachment to the free margin of the gingiva. During this exploratory stroke, the tip or blade will become caught or will "bump over" large pieces or ledges of calculus. "Dragging" or "sticking" of the working end is perceived as the instrument rubs over smaller pieces or sheets of calculus. Roughened cementum or an irregular cemento-enamel junction may also convey this "sticky" feeling. A clean enamel or cemental surface should feel completely smooth—almost glass-like. You will be able to feel and develop your own favorite adjectives for these sensations.

Working Stroke. When the curette or any other scaling instrument encounters a piece of calculus or an irregularity in the root surface, a working stroke is employed to remove the deposit and smooth the root surface. The *grasp is tightened,* and *more pressure is applied* to the tooth surface to enable clean removal of the deposit by the blade. The working stroke is drawn from the area just beneath the deposit to the free margin of the gingiva. After the deposit has been dislodged, the blade should be reinserted and an exploratory stroke should be used in the same area to evaluate the success of the working stroke.

The *pull stroke* is more widely used and much safer than the *push stroke*. Even when used by an experienced operator, the push stroke may detach or tear the epithelial attachment and embed fragments of crushed calculus and debris into the sulcular epithelium. Therefore, the push stroke is not recommended for calculus removal.

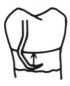

Vertical Stroke

Oblique Stroke

Horizontal Stroke

Exploratory and working strokes may be directed vertically, obliquely, or horizontally. *Vertical strokes* are most effective because they are directed in the same plane as the long axis of the tooth. If you recall your dental anatomy, you know that the tooth surface feels fairly regular when you draw an instrument up and down on a tooth. If you try to draw the instrument around horizontally or circumferentially, you discover that there are numerous line angles, grooves, and furcations that make angulation and adaptation much more difficult. Of course, in some areas, such as the line angles of molars, vertical strokes are quite difficult to achieve. The *oblique stroke* is also very effective and should be used in such cases. It is very easy to succumb to the habit of constantly using a *horizontal stroke,* but as the illustration above shows, this stroke is hazardous to the epithelial attachment and is also the most ineffective of the three strokes.

The muscles of the upper arm and shoulder, the forearm, wrist, hand, and fingers all contribute to the activation of strokes during instrumentation. It is important that the wrist and forearm be the prime movers, however, because heavy dependence upon the muscles of the fingers will result in cramping and less efficient removal of calculus. Watch your fingers as you activate strokes to make sure that you are not pushing and pulling on the instrument with your fingers alone. Always try to use your wrist, forearm, and shoulder and take full advantage of your finger rest. By developing good habits and good body mechanics now, you will avoid suffering the pain of muscle fatigue after a day in the clinic or on the job.

It is important to note that during any exploratory or working stroke, *maximum tactile sensitivity is gained when as much of the working end or cutting edge as possible is in contact with the tooth or deposit.* When using the curette, students often try to remove calculus with the toe of the instrument rather than the length of the cutting edge. Watch your angulation and anticipate the convexities and concavities in the tooth surface by recalling your knowledge of dental anatomy, especially root morphology.

Another important factor influencing the complete removal of calculus is the *extension of strokes into interproximal areas.* When scaling a proximal surface such as the mesial or distal of a molar, be sure to extend strokes at least halfway across the surface when you approach from both the buccal and lingual sides to insure complete removal of interproximal deposits. This is critical when using the explorer since much calculus is left in these areas simply because it is not detected by the explorer before or after scaling.

ACTIVATING EXPLORATORY STROKES: EXPLORER ON EXTRACTED TOOTH

Let's begin by doing some exploratory strokes with the explorer on an extracted molar that has calculus on its root surfaces. This is the only type of stroke to be used with the explorer since it is a detection instrument, rather than a scaling instrument with cutting edges. As you activate these strokes, remember to hold the handle with a light grasp and gently rub the explorer tip against the tooth surface. Pay particular attention to the textures and sensations you feel as the tip encounters pieces of calculus of different shapes, sizes, and consistencies. Take time to feel clean, smooth enamel and cementum, irregular or rough cementum, and any defects in the root surfaces. Compare these areas with the calculus, first with your eyes open, and then with your eyes closed.

Do not be too discouraged if you have difficulty distinguishing anything other than very smooth enamel or very obvious rough calculus. Good tactile sensitivity is learned only through extended practice. We all rely so heavily on our visual senses that few of us are able to feel such slight surface variations through our fingers. Perhaps dental hygienists could learn a great deal from the blind, who are particularly gifted in this skill.

Use your pencil to mark an imaginary epithelial attachment on the mounted extracted molar that has calculus on its root surfaces. Witnessing how far apically the attachment has migrated on heavily encrusted teeth is vividly educational as well as alarming.

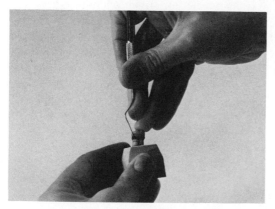

1. Grasp the explorer and establish your occlusal finger rest. Adapt the tip to the buccal surface of the tooth at the distal line angle with the tip directed mesially.

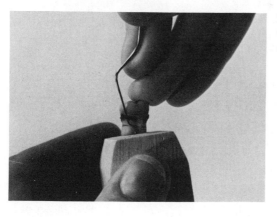

2. Insert the explorer to the epithelial attachment according to all previous instructions.

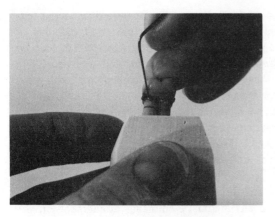

3. Begin activating continuous, short, overlapping, vertical or oblique strokes by rotating your wrist and forearm slightly from left to right, pivoting on your finger rest.

Use exploratory strokes across the buccal surface of the molar. Extend each stroke from the epithelial attachment to the approximate location of the free margin of the gingiva.

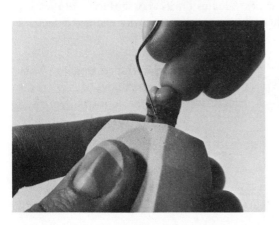

4. As you approach the mesial line angle, rotate the wrist from right to left and roll the handle from right to left in your fingers to keep the sharp point constantly in contact with the tooth surface while you are adapting the tip. A common error with the use of the explorer is to use only the side of the tip. This allows the point no longer in contact with the tooth to lacerate tissue and also minimizes tactile sensitivity.

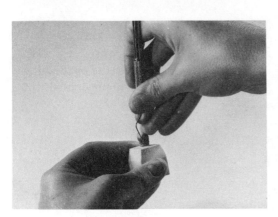

5. Continue to activate strokes across the mesial surface by lifting your wrist and rocking forward on your finger rest. Be sure to keep the tip against the tooth during the entire stroke. Extend strokes at least halfway across the mesial surface.

After exploring the buccal and mesial surfaces, carefully withdraw the tip from the sulcus.

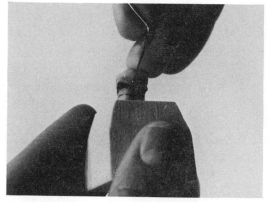

6. To explore the distal surface, adapt the tip to the buccal surface with the tip again directed distally.

Reinsert the tip at a position slightly mesial to the distal line angle.

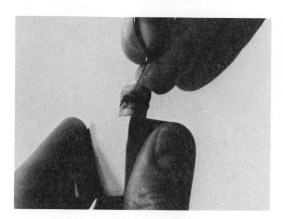

7. Activate exploratory strokes by rotating your wrist from left to right. Remember also to roll the handle from left to right in your fingers as you use strokes around the distal line angle.

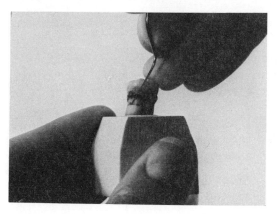

8. Keep activating *short, overlapping* strokes across the distal surface by rotating your wrist from left to right, pivoting on your finger rest. Extend strokes at least halfway across the distal surface.

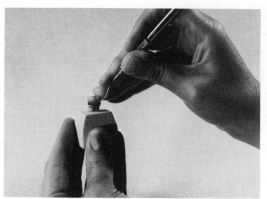

9. Exploring the distal surfaces of the molars in the mouth is difficult because the cheek limits access from the buccal aspect. Therefore, strokes activated by lowering the wrist and rocking back on the finger rest are easier to accomplish and more effective.

Again, extend strokes at least halfway across the distal surface.

Now that you know how to activate an exploratory stroke, turn the molar around and explore away! Work on several other extracted molars that have calculus to gain as much experience as possible in tactile discrimination. Lead your explorer tip on an adventurous trek over calculus ledges and rough cementum, across developmental grooves, into the depths of furcations, and finish it off with a leisurely trip along the cemento-enamel junction! It is wise to become familiar with the CEJ by using short, exploratory strokes over it all the way around the tooth. That slight lump which marks the transition from cementum to enamel is one of the great deceivers. Students have been known to explore and scale such lumps for endless periods to no avail. Concentrated practice and good recall of dental anatomy should spare you this common frustration.

Activating Exploratory Strokes: Explorer on Manikin

Let's repeat this exercise on the manikin now. This time there's an interesting challenge involved. Artificial calculus has been randomly applied to the teeth of the manikin; and now we'll see if you can find it!

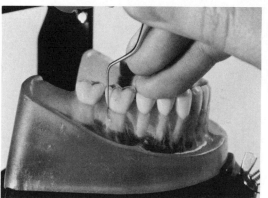

1. Grasp the explorer and establish a finger rest on the occlusal surfaces of the mandibular right bicuspids.

Adapt the tip at the distal line angle and insert to the epithelial attachment.

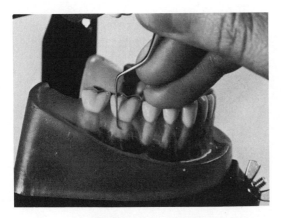

2. Activate exploratory strokes across the buccal surface by rotating your wrist slightly from left to right or by lowering your wrist and rocking back on your finger rest.

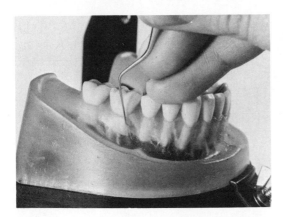

3. As you approach the mesial line angle, roll the handle from left to right in your fingers to keep the tip constantly adapted to the tooth surface.

Note: The ability to roll the instrument around the line angles is the key to successful scaling. This technique minimizes the chances of trauma and optimizes the proficiency of scaling.

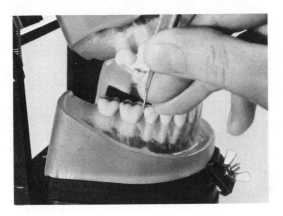

4. Lower your wrist and rock back on your finger rest to activate strokes across the mesial surface. Continue at least halfway across the mesial surface.

After exploring the buccal and mesial surfaces, carefully withdraw the tip from the sulcus.

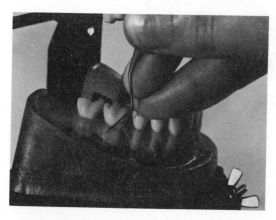

5. Adapt the tip to the buccal surface of the tooth again, with the tip directed distally this time.

Reinsert the tip at a position slightly mesial to the distal line angle.

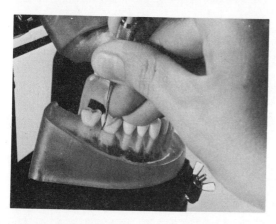

6. Activate exploratory strokes by rotating your wrist from left to right. Remember to rotate the handle from left to right in your fingers as you use strokes around the distal line angle.

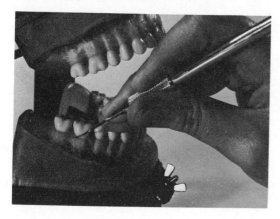

7. On the distal surface, activate strokes by lowering the wrist and rocking back on the finger rest.

Extend strokes at least halfway across the distal surface.

Continue to explore the second and first bicuspids in the same manner.

Review Questions for Lesson F: Activating a Stroke

Read the following statements before answering the first two questions.
　　1. The handle is grasped lightly.
　　2. The handle is grasped very firmly.
　　3. Light pressure is applied to the tooth surface.
　　4. Firm pressure is applied to the tooth surface.
　　5. Stroke extends from area just beneath deposit to free margin.
　　6. Stroke extends from epithelial attachment to free margin.

1. Which of the above statements describe the exploratory stroke?
　　a. 1,3,5
　　b. 1,4,6
　　c. 2,4,5
　　d. 1,3,6

2. Which of the above statements describe the working stroke?
　　a. 1,4,5
　　b. 1,4,6
　　c. 2,4,5
　　d. 2,3,6

3. Heavy dependence upon muscles of the fingers during activation of strokes will result in:
　　a. cramping and fatigue
　　b. more efficient removal of calculus
　　c. good body mechanics
　　d. better tactile sensitivity

4. For complete removal of calculus on a proximal surface, strokes should be extended:
　　a. to the cemento-enamel junction
　　b. just under the gingiva
　　c. onto the lingual surface
　　d. at least halfway across the surface

5. Keeping as much of the working end or cutting edge as possible in contact with the tooth or deposit will result in:
　　a. maximum tactile sensitivity
　　b. effective calculus removal
　　c. laceration of tissue with the toe
　　d. all of the above
　　e. a and b only

Read the following phrases before answering the next four questions.
　　1. Likely to injure the epithelial attachment
　　2. Directed in same plane as long axis of tooth
　　3. Directed circumferentially around tooth
　　4. When vertical strokes are difficult, good for posterior teeth
　　5. Embeds fragments of calculus into the sulcular epithelium

6. Which of the above phrases apply to the push stroke?
　　a. 1,4
　　b. 1,5

    c. 2,4

    d. 5 only

7. Which of the above phrases apply to the vertical stroke?

    a. 2 only

    b. 1,3

    c. 2,4

    d. 5 only

8. Which of the above phrases apply to the oblique stroke?

    a. 1,4

    b. 3 only

    c. 4 only

    d. 3,4

9. Which of the above phrases apply to the horizontal stroke?

    a. 1,2

    b. 1,3

    c. 1,3,4

    d. 2,5

Correct your answers with the Answer Key on page 73.

Performance Checklist for Lesson F: Activating a Stroke

Name ————————————

School ———————————

Date ————————————

		#1		#2	
		SATISFACTORY	UNSATISFACTORY	SATISFACTORY	UNSATISFACTORY
16.	Demonstrate exploratory strokes with the explorer on an extracted molar.				
17.	Describe how subgingival calculus on extracted teeth feels when using exploratory strokes with the explorer.				
18.	Demonstrate exploratory strokes with the explorer on the manikin's mandibular right first molar, second bicuspid and first bicuspid.				
19.	Locate all artifical subgingival and supragingival calculus on the distal, buccal, and mesial surfaces of these three teeth.				

Instructor ————————————

Performance Check Time ————————————

Comments: ————————————————

————————————————————

————————————————————

————————————————————

ACTIVATING EXPLORATORY STROKES: CURETTE ON EXTRACTED TOOTH

The principles of activating exploratory strokes with the curette are almost the same as those for the explorer. This stroke is used interchangeably with the working stroke during scaling. The curette is drawn gently over the tooth surface at working angulation to locate calculus. If calculus is encountered, the grasp is tightened and a series of working strokes is employed.

As you work with the curette on the extracted molars, try to describe the textures that you feel. Make sure that you feel all of the deposits and surfaces that you felt with the explorer. See if the curette increases or diminishes your tactile sensitivity. Decide whether the explorer or the curette should be the "final judge" in determining complete removal of calculus.

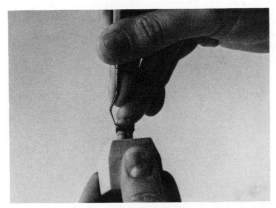

1. Grasp the curette and establish your occlusal finger rest. Adapt the blade to the buccal surface of the molar at the distal line angle. Direct the blade mesially and check the position of the face of the blade to make sure you are working with the correct end of the curette.

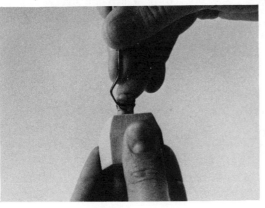

2. Insert the curette to the epithelial attachment, according to previous instructions.

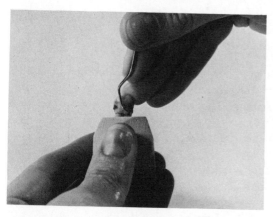

3. Begin activating exploratory strokes across the buccal surface by rotating your wrist and forearm slightly from left to right.

Remember to hold the handle lightly, but securely, and to try to develop the "sight" in your fingers by closing your eyes periodically.

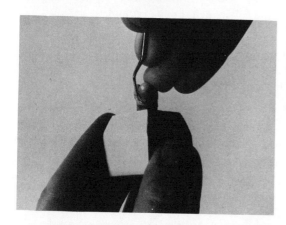

4. As you approach the mesial line angle, roll the handle from left to right in your fingers to *keep the blade constantly adapted to the tooth surface.* Adjust blade angulation to compensate for the natural curvatures in the tooth surface.

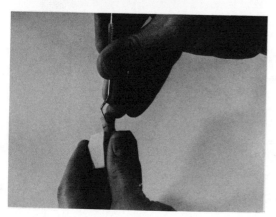

5. Lift your wrist and rock forward on your finger rest to activate strokes across the mesial surface. Continue all the way across the mesial surface.

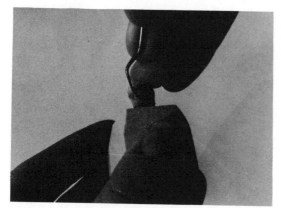

6. Turn the extracted molar around so that its lingual surface is toward you. Continue exploratory strokes across the lingual and distal surfaces of the tooth. By turning the tooth you will be able to feel all surfaces without changing ends of the curette.

ACTIVATING WORKING STROKES: CURETTE ON EXTRACTED TOOTH

Now that you have learned to use an exploratory stroke with the curette, repeat the exercise once more, but this time try using a working stroke whenever you encounter calculus or rough cementum. Tighten your grasp, make sure you have established good working angulation, and remove the deposit with firm, overlapping, vertical or oblique strokes until you have created a smooth, clean surface.

For this particular lesson you must reserve one extracted molar to be used later during your performance check. Practice working strokes on all but one of the molars, removing all calculus and smoothing the root surfaces. Feel the root surfaces with the explorer after you have completed the scaling on each tooth.

ACTIVATING EXPLORATORY STROKES: CURETTE ON MANIKIN

Now let's move on to an exploratory stroke exercise on the manikin. You will work on the mandibular right first molar, second bicuspid, and first bicuspid, feeling only the buccal and mesial surfaces of each tooth. Although you felt the distal surfaces of these teeth with the explorer, selection of the working end and specific cutting edge may vary for the distal surfaces of molars when using the curette.

This technique will be taught in Module III (The Removal of Light to Moderate Calculus); we will not get involved in an explanation of it now. All you need be concerned with at this time is the nature of the exploratory and the working stroke. You can accomplish this quite satisfactorily by *limiting your instrumentation to the buccal and mesial surfaces of these three teeth.*

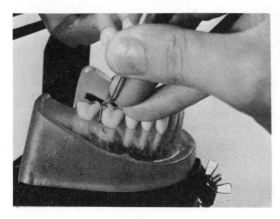

1. Grasp the curette and establish a finger rest on the occlusal surfaces of the mandibular right bicuspids.

Select the correct end of the curette, place the blade on the first molar at the distal line angle, and insert it to the epithelial attachment.

Lift the handle so the toe of the curette is not pointing down toward the epithelial attachment.

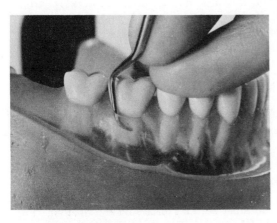

2. Activate exploratory strokes across the buccal surface by rotating your wrist slightly from left to right.

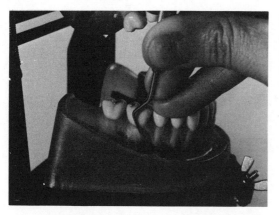

3. As you approach the mesial line angle, rotate the handle from left to right in your fingers to keep the blade constantly adapted to the tooth surface.

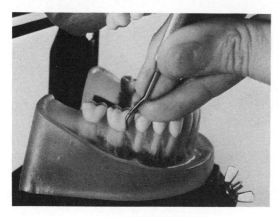

4. Lower your wrist and rock back on your finger rest to activate strokes across the mesial surface. Extend strokes at least halfway across the mesial surface.

Withdraw the curette blade from the sulcus by gently drawing the blade up and away from the interproximal area. Be careful not to let the blade become lodged in the contact point.

Move on to the second and first bicuspids. Use exploratory strokes on the buccal and mesial surfaces only.

Did you feel the artificial calculus with the curette as well as you did with the explorer? The fine sensitivity achieved with the explorer explains why the explorer should always be used to determine whether removal of calculus is complete.

Review Questions for Lesson F: Activating a Stroke (cont.)

10. Number the following steps in the order in which they should be performed:
   _____ Tighten grasp
   _____ Create a smooth surface
   _____ Use exploratory strokes with curette
   _____ Activate a series of working strokes
   _____ Locate calculus
   _____ Remove all calculus
   _____ Check surface with explorer and rescale if necessary

11. While activating the curette, the exploratory stroke is used:
    a. only after removal of calculus
    b. very seldom
    c. interchangeably with the working stroke
    d. exclusively

12. Which instrument should always be used as the "final judge" to determine whether removal of calculus has been completed? Why?

Correct your answers with the Answer Key on page 73.

Performance Checklist for Lesson F: Activating a Stroke (Cont.)

Name _____

School _____

Date _____

	#1		#2	
	SATISFACTORY	UNSATISFACTORY	SATISFACTORY	UNSATISFACTORY
20. Demonstrate exploratory strokes with the curette on an extracted molar.				
21. Describe how subgingival calculus on extracted teeth feels when using exploratory strokes with the curette.				
22. Demonstrate exploratory strokes with the curette on the manikin's mandibular right first molar, second bicuspid, and first bicuspid.				
23. Locate all artificial subgingival and supragingival calculus on only the buccal and mesial surfaces of these three teeth.				

Instructor _____

Performance Check Time _____

Comments: _____

_____

_____

_____

ACTIVATING WORKING STROKES: CURETTE ON MANIKIN

Now that you are ready to begin using working strokes on the manikin, you should be made aware of another common difficulty. Contact points in interproximal areas present a problem to many beginning students. Curette blades invariably become caught in contacts when strokes are extended too far coronally. You may avoid this difficulty by using careful, short strokes that stop just short of the contact point. A forceful, sweeping stroke into the contact often causes the student to react with sheer panic. Tugging, wrenching, or yanking the instrument only complicates matters by increasing the chances for breakage of the tip. This struggling also creates a genuine feeling of apprehension in the patient.

The simplest solution to this problem is to loosen your grasp on the instrument, apply no pressure, move the handle up and down with a slight vertical motion, and let the weight of the instrument pull the tip free. As you perform the working stroke exercises on the manikin, try this rescue procedure whenever you find yourself in such a "bind."

Work on the mandibular right first molar, second bicuspid, and first bicuspid as you did before, and remove all the artificial calculus on the buccal and mesial surfaces only. Check all three teeth carefully with the explorer for residual deposits and rescale where necessary.

Review Questions for Lesson F: Activating a Stroke (cont.)

13. Curette blades become caught in contact points when strokes are extended:
    a. too far periodontally
    b. too far coronally
    c. too far apically
    d. too far subgingivally

14. If this problem occurs, it is best solved by:
    a. moving the handle up and down slightly
    b. using careful strokes which stop short of the contact
    c. tightening your grasp on the instrument
    d. applying more pressure against the tooth

Correct your answers with the Answer Key on page 73.

Name _____

School _____

Date _____

		#1			#2	
		SATISFACTORY	UNSATISFACTORY		SATISFACTORY	UNSATISFACTORY
24.	Demonstrate working strokes with the curette on an extracted molar.					
25.	Remove all subgingival calculus from an extracted molar using working strokes with the curette.					
26.	Demonstrate working strokes with the curette on the manikin's mandibular right first molar, second bicuspid, and first bicuspid.					
27.	Remove all artificial subgingival and supragingival calculus from the buccal and mesial surfaces of these three teeth with the curette.*					

Instructor _____

Performance Check Time _____

Comments: _____

_____

_____

_____

* Upon completion of your performance check, remove the three teeth from the manikin and examine them with your instructor. How did you do? If there is any residual calculus, can you determine why you missed it?

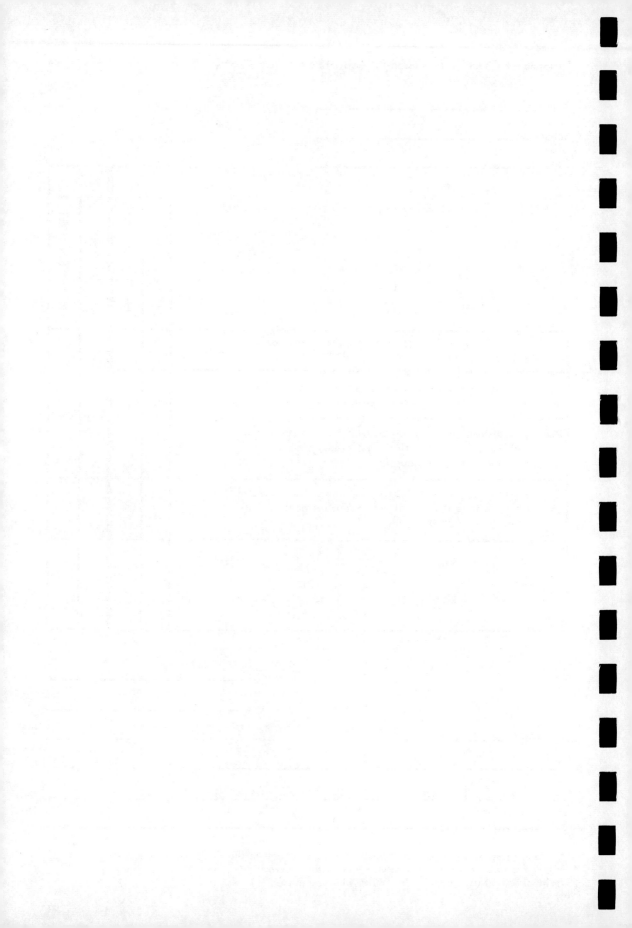

CONGRATULATIONS!
YOU HAVE NOW MASTERED THE FUNDAMENTAL SKILLS
FOR INSTRUMENTATION.

If you are interested in reading more about fundamental skills, refer to the "Reading Assignments for Enrichment" on page 74.

FINGER REST EXERCISES

The following exercises will help you to establish good intraoral finger rests. They will give you practice in the three important wrist-arm movements, which you will use to activate your instruments. Notice the importance of the ring finger as a "pivoting point" as you perform these exercises.

EXERCISE A

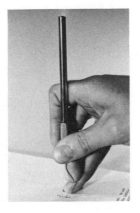

1. Hold the explorer with a modified pen grasp and place the pad of your ring finger on the circle below the photograph. Do not rest any other part of your hand or arm on the desk. Grasp the explorer close to the working end and position the handle so it is perpendicular to the paper. Keep your wrist and elbow up so they are level with your hand or elevated slightly above it. The side of your middle finger should be resting against the side of your ring finger, as shown.

2. Place the tip of the explorer on the upper end of the dotted line. Rotate your wrist and forearm very slightly from left to right until you have lifted the tip about an eighth of an inch off the paper. Repeat this motion several times so that you are rocking on your finger rest and "walking" the tip down the dotted line.

Try this exercise again, but this time do not use a finger rest. Do not rest any part of your hand or arm on the desk. Can you lift the instrument tip just an eighth of an inch and follow the dotted line with accuracy? Does your hand feel as steady as it did when you used a finger rest?

EXERCISE B

Place the pad of your ring finger in the circle as in Exercise A. Place the end of the explorer on the dot with the tip pointing in the direction of the arrow. The explorer handle should be perpendicular to the paper and your arm should not be resting on the desk.

Now rock back on your finger rest by lowering your wrist and arm. Continue rocking on your finger rest by lifting and lowering your wrist. The explorer tip should be moving straight up and down along the solid line.

EXERCISE C

Place the pad of your ring finger in the circle and the end of your explorer on the dot as in Exercise B. The tip should be pointing in the direction of the arrow. Make sure the handle is perpendicular to the paper.

Lift your wrist and arm so that you are rocking forward on your finger rest. Keep rocking forward and backward so that the tip moves up and down along the solid line.

ANSWER KEY

LESSON A

1. a—working end
   b—shank
   c—handle
2. b
3. a—curette
   b—Columbia
   c—Star Dental Company
   d—13-14

   e—double
4. d
5. g
6. e
7. c
8. c
9. c

LESSON B

1. d
2. a
3. modified pen
4. b
5. b
6. c

LESSON C

1. ring
2. d
3. b
4. The intraoral finger rest is safer because it is established on a firm, stable surface. The extraoral finger rest is less stable because the skin is supple; therefore there is greater danger of slipping and injuring the patient.

LESSON D

1. parallel
2. a
3. a
4. b
5.

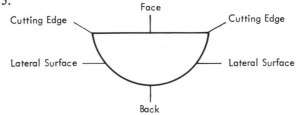

LESSON D (continued)

6. d
7. a
8. b

LESSON E

1. d
2. b
3. a
4. b
5. c
6. b

LESSON F

1. d
2. c
3. a
4. d
5. e
6. b
7. a
8. c
9. b
10. a—3
    b—6
    c—1
    d—4
    e—2
    f—5
    g—7
11. c
12. The explorer should be used as the "final judge" because it allows better tactile sensitivity than the curette or any other calculus removal instruments.
13. b
14. a

READING ASSIGNMENTS FOR REVIEW *

1. *Patient and Operator Positioning:*
   Wilkins, *Clinical Practice of the Dental Hygienist*, pp. 35–42.
   Steele, *Dimensions of Dental Hygiene*, pp. 158–162.

2. *Oral Anatomy:*
   Wilkins, *Clinical Practice of the Dental Hygienist*, pp. 110–118.
   Steele, *Dimensions of Dental Hygiene*, pp. 55–69.

3. *Dental Anatomy:*
   Steele, *Dimensions of Dental Hygiene*, pp. 70–83, 83–101 (root morphology only)
   Wheeler, *A Textbook of Dental Anatomy and Physiology*, pp. 3–15.

4. *Introduction to the Oral Prophylaxis:*
   Wilkins, *Clinical Practice of the Dental Hygienist*, pp. 3–6, 143–149.
   Steele, *Dimensions of Dental Hygiene*, pp. 15–33, 145.

READING ASSIGNMENTS FOR ENRICHMENT *

Steele, *Dimensions of Dental Hygiene*, pp. 158–183 (Oral Prophylaxis)
Wilkins, *Clinical Practice of the Dental Hygienist:*
   pp. 150–162 (Soft Deposits and Dental Calculus)
   pp. 171–177 (Principles of Technique for Oral Prophylaxis)
   pp. 180–185 (Instruments and Sharpening)
   pp. 197–208 (Scaling and Root Planing)
Goldman and Cohen, *Periodontal Therapy:*
   pp. 209–264 (Etiology)
   pp. 336–347 (Rationale for Periodontal Therapy)
   pp. 389–404 (Instrumentation for Scaling and Root Planing)
   pp. 405–445 (Scaling and Root Planing)

* See bibliography on page 252 for complete identification of publications listed here.
* See bibliography on page 252 for complete identification of publications listed here.

MODULE II

The Detection
of Calculus
and
Periodontal Pockets

1. PREREQUISITES

Before beginning work on this module, you must have successfully completed Module I. You will encounter difficulty in understanding instructions and performing the skills throughout this module if you have not passed all of the performance checks in Module I.

In addition to completion of Module I, a review of patient and operator positioning is recommended as well as knowledge in the following areas:

A. STERILIZATION, DISINFECTION, AND SANITIZATION

1) transmission of disease
2) handwashing
3) sterilization of instruments
4) sanitization of the dental unit

B. Introduction to Periodontics

1) etiology of periodontal disease
2) introduction to the periodontal disease process
3) formation and attachment of plaque and calculus

If some review is needed in any of these areas, turn to page 159 and read the suggested assignment for the particular subject. If you are then confident of your knowledge, proceed with the module.

2. PERFORMANCE OBJECTIVES

A. General Objective

Given a mirror, explorer, periodontal probe, air syringe, and a fellow-student patient, the student will be able to demonstrate the procedure for the detection of calculus and periodontal pockets. Also, given a full mouth set of radiographs, the student will be able to detect all calculus that is evident in the radiographs.

B. Specific Objectives

Without the aid of source materials, the student will be able to:

1) demonstrate the appropriate fulcrums for the mirror and explorer in the following twelve areas of the mouth:

a) Mandibular Right Posterior—Buccal Aspect
b) Mandibular Right Posterior—Lingual Aspect
c) Mandibular Anterior—Labial Aspect
d) Mandibular Anterior—Lingual Aspect
e) Mandibular Left Posterior—Buccal Aspect
f) Mandibular Left Posterior—Lingual Aspect
g) Maxillary Right Posterior—Buccal Aspect
h) Maxillary Right Posterior—Lingual Aspect
i) Maxillary Anterior—Labial Aspect
j) Maxillary Anterior—Lingual Aspect
k) Maxillary Left Posterior—Buccal Aspect
l) Maxillary Left Posterior—Lingual Aspect

2) demonstrate the use of the mirror and explorer for calculus detection in these areas.

3) demonstrate the use of the periodontal probe to measure six

specific areas (disto-buccal, buccal, mesio-buccal, disto-lingual, lingual, and mesio-lingual) on a molar of a fellow-student patient or manikin.

4) demonstrate the use of the periodontal probe to measure these same six areas on an anterior tooth of a fellow-student patient or manikin.

5) demonstrate the use of compressed air on the lingual aspect of the mandibular anterior teeth to detect supragingival calculus on a fellow-student patient.

6) demonstrate the use of compressed air to deflect the gingiva on a fellow-student patient.

7) examine a full mouth set of radiographs and detect all evident calculus.

3. DIRECTIONS FOR THE USE OF THE MODULE

The following materials and equipment are required for the successful completion of this module:

    a dental mirror
    an explorer
    a periodontal probe
    an air syringe
    *a full mouth set of radiographs
    a dental manikin or a fellow-student patient

If you are going to work on a fellow-student patient, make sure that all of your instruments have been sterilized. When you are ready to perform the step-by-step procedures, have your patient hold up the copy of the module for you so that you can read the steps and refer to the photographs as you work in her mouth. If you are working on a manikin, set it up at your lab station and place the instruments on the desk next to the module.

After you have finished reading the Skills Lesson, answer the review questions, and verify them with the Answer Key. When you have answered all of the questions correctly and have practiced the skill sufficiently, ask your instructor for a performance check. If your instructor is occupied and cannot check you immediately, you may go on to the next lesson while you are waiting. As you demonstrate your skill, the instructor will record your performance as satisfactory or unsatisfactory. If your ratings are all satisfactory, proceed to the next Skills Lesson. If any of your ratings are unsatisfactory, review the exercises and request a second performance check when you are ready.

* This item will be provided by the instructor.

4. SKILLS LESSONS

Lesson A: *Detecting Calculus with the Mirror and Explorer*

In addition to the instruments used to remove calculus, there are two that are absolutely essential for scaling procedures: the mirror and the explorer. Without these aids, it is impossible to perform a thorough prophylaxis.

Mirror. The mirror is used to obtain indirect vision, illumination, transillumination, and retraction, all of which allow more proficient examination of supragingival calculus and periodontal tissues. There are many areas of the mouth where direct vision is either impaired or impossible during instrumentation. For example, the lingual surfaces of the maxillary anterior teeth demand the use of indirect vision; therefore, in that area you must learn to work by observing images in the mirror. The mirror provides *illumination* (the addition of light to an area by reflection of the mirror), and *transillumination* (the reflection of light from the lingual aspect through the teeth as they are examined from a buccal aspect). The mirror accomplishes this by reflecting a beam of light from the dental unit lamp onto the surface to be viewed. This technique is used to detect caries, supragingival calculus, and to a lesser extent, subgingival calculus. The mirror is also used to retract the cheeks, lips, and tongue for better access and illumination. It is important to remember that the mirror is best utilized when its functions are combined and employed simultaneously, e.g., when it is used for both indirect vision and illumination.

The mirror has three parts: the handle, the shank, and the working end or mirror head. Mirror heads vary in size from ⅝ inch to 1¼ inch in diameter. The face or reflecting surface of the mirror is the most important feature to consider in selecting a mirror. The types of faces to choose from are: plane (flat), magnifying (concave), or front-surface (reflecting surface on front rather than back). The plane surface mirror is difficult to use because it reflects a double image. The front-surface mirror does not have this disadvantage and is the type most commonly used by dental hygienists. Mirror handles should be large enough to allow a comfortable modified pen grasp.

Explorer. The explorer is used to detect supragingival calculus, subgingival calculus, caries, decalcification, abnormalities in tooth morphology, irregularities in cemental surfaces, and to examine the contours of dental restorations. The explorer is a flexible, wire-like instrument, which is circular in cross section and ends in a sharp point. The extreme end of the explorer is referred to as the *point,* and the terminal 1 to 2 mm of the working end behind the point is called the *tip*. The explorer is the most sensitive tool for detection because its fine structure allows vibrations to be transmitted through the handle as subtle surface irregularities are encountered.

Explorers are manufactured in a variety of shapes and sizes. They may be single-ended, double-ended with paired working ends, or double-ended with dissimilar working ends. The illustrations below show some of the more commonly used types of explorers.

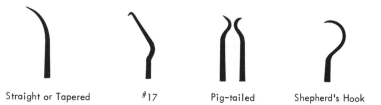

| Straight or Tapered | #17 | Pig-tailed | Shepherd's Hook |

The straight or tapered explorer is utilized for detection of calculus and caries. Be sure to examine the working end very carefully when selecting this type of explorer because it is often too thick to allow optimal tactile sensitivity and subgingival adaptation to the tooth surface. As with all other explorers, the tip must be very fine in order to evaluate completion of scaling and root planing.

The #17 explorer is used primarily for calculus detection. The fine 2 mm tip, which is at right angles to the shank, is excellent for detection of calculus in deep pockets and furcations. Good adaptation of this instrument is imperative because of the right-angled tip, especially on curved surfaces such as the line angles.

Pig-tailed explorers must be paired, whether they are single- or double-ended. These explorers are easily adapted to most surfaces, but they are not suitable for deep pockets and furcations. They are generally very thin and therefore provide good tactile sensitivity. They are also very good for caries detection.

The shepherd's hook explorer is reserved primarily for detection of caries and supragingival calculus. It is usually too thick for good tactile sensitivity, and its design prohibits good adaptation in interproximal areas. Exploration of furcations and deep pockets is not recommended with this type of explorer.

When selecting an appropriate explorer, look for versatility, adaptability, and sensitivity. Selection is obviously dictated by the specific use you have in mind.

Hold the explorer with a light but firm modified pen grasp. Activate light exploratory strokes using the tip of the explorer, rather than the point, to feel each surface. You discovered in Module I that concentration is a very important factor in exploring technique. As an extension of your tactile sense, the explorer is capable of encountering irregularities, but only you can interpret what you feel, and only you can distinguish calculus, cementum, the cemento-enamel junction (CEJ), and other structures from each other.

Use the explorer for initial examination to determine the location and amount of subgingival calculus prior to scaling and root planing. Be sure to check carefully with the mirror and explorer throughout the prophylaxis, and especially during definitive scaling and root planing, to insure complete removal of deposits and stains. *Remember that the explorer is the most sensitive instrument you possess* and should be used in your final evaluation of the prophylaxis.

Having completed Module I, you should be well acquainted with the modified pen grasp, finger rests, insertion, adaptation, and activation of exploratory strokes. Now you are ready to learn to use the mirror and the explorer in all of the different areas of the mouth. Apply the principles and techniques you have learned as you perform this exercise on a fellow-student patient or a manikin.

If you are working on a fellow-student patient, remember that your instruments must be sterile before you perform this exercise. Be sure to wash your hands before beginning work in the mouth and maintain the chain of asepsis as you work. You will begin exploring on the buccal aspect of the mandibular right posterior teeth because this is the area in which you have practiced previously. The order of instrumentation in this exercise represents only one of many possible sequences. Your instructor should indicate the order of instrumentation that is taught in your particular school. Also, in those areas where several finger rests are shown, your instructor may indicate the ones that are preferred. *Remember that there is no one absolute technique for instrumentation;* there are many variations, and you will often encounter strong regional or personal preferences. Keep in mind that the best techniques are those that are comfortable, efficient, and effective for both you and your patient.

There are six performance checks for this exercise.* After using the mirror and explorer on the facial and lingual surfaces of any given area, you must stop and request a performance check before moving on to the next area. These frequent checks will help to prevent your making the same mistakes on more than one area.

* There is only one set of review questions for all six Performance Checks in Lesson A. It can be found at the end of the lesson, on page 133.

MANDIBULAR RIGHT POSTERIOR TEETH (#32–#28)

Buccal Aspect

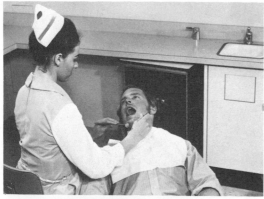

1. You should be positioned at the side of the patient. His mouth should be level with or lower than your elbow. The headrest and backrest should be positioned so that the patient's neck and spine are in a straight line.

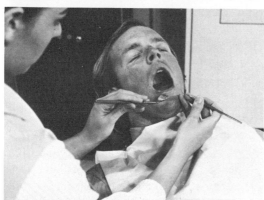

2. Tell the patient to turn his head slightly away from you. This position allows maximum direct vision. Instructions to the patient should always be polite verbal commands. Do not turn the patient's head with your hands because this would break the chain of asepsis and you would have to rewash your hands.

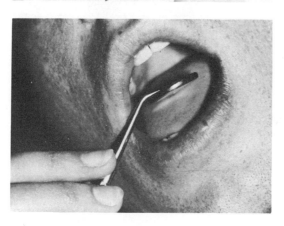

3. Pick up the mirror with your left hand. Insert the mirror head so that it is parallel to the occlusal plane. Then move the mirror laterally to the buccal mucosa.

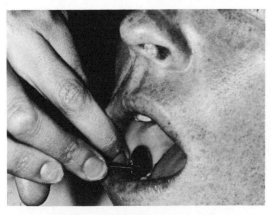

4. Use direct vision in this area with the mirror retracting the buccal mucosa. Your mirror finger rest may be established by:

a. Placing the ring finger on the buccal mucosa and gently pulling the cheek away from the teeth.

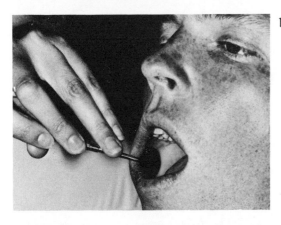

b. Placing the ring finger on the shank of the mirror and then gently pulling the cheek away from the teeth.

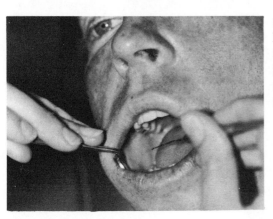

5. Pick up the explorer with your right hand. Carefully insert the explorer into the mouth. Make sure the patient's mouth is open wide enough so that you do not touch the lips or any oral structures with the sharp tip.

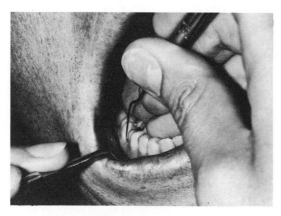

6. Establish your instrument finger rest by placing your ring finger on the occlusal surfaces of the teeth closest to your working area.

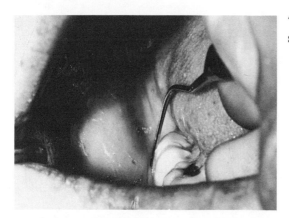

7. Begin exploring the buccal and mesial surfaces of the posterior-most molar.

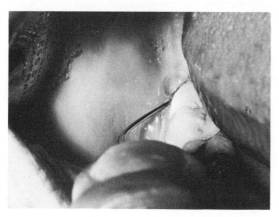

8. Then explore the distal surface of this tooth.

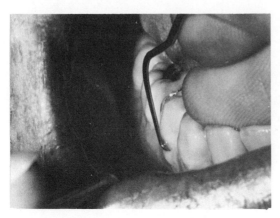

9. Move on to the buccal and mesial surfaces and then the distal surface of the next tooth. Continue exploring each tooth in this manner from the last tooth in the quadrant to the first bicuspid.

MANDIBULAR RIGHT POSTERIOR TEETH (#32–#28)

LINGUAL ASPECT

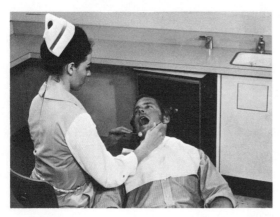

1. Position yourself at the side of the patient.

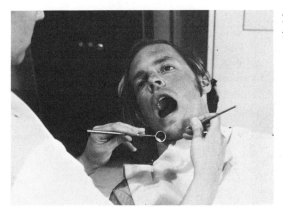

2. Direct the patient to turn his head toward you.

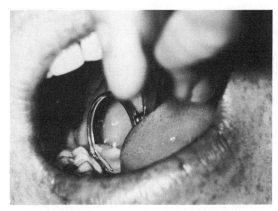

3. Pick up the mirror with your left hand and establish a finger rest on the labial surface of the maxillary left cuspid area. Use direct vision if possible, with the mirror retracting the tongue and reflecting light. If you cannot have direct vision, use the mirror for indirect vision, retraction of the tongue, and reflection of light on the working area.

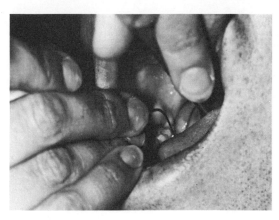

4. Your instrument finger rest should be on the occlusal surfaces of the mandibular right bicuspids.

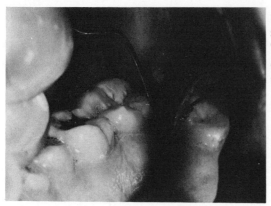

5. Begin exploring the lingual and mesial surfaces of the posterior-most molar. Then explore the distal surface and proceed to the next tooth. Continue forward to the first bicuspid.

When you think you have practiced exploring this area sufficiently and are confident of your technique, request a performance check.

Performance Checklist for Lesson A: Detecting Calculus with the Mirror and Explorer

Name _____

School _____

Date _____

	#1		#2	
	SATISFACTORY	UNSATISFACTORY	SATISFACTORY	UNSATISFACTORY
1. Demonstrate the appropriate FULCRUMS for the mirror and explorer on the BUCCAL aspect of the MANDIBULAR RIGHT POSTERIOR teeth.				
2. Demonstrate the USE of the mirror and explorer for calculus detection on the BUCCAL aspect of the MANDIBULAR RIGHT POSTERIOR teeth.				
3. Demonstrate the appropriate FULCRUMS for the mirror and explorer on the LINGUAL aspect of the MANDIBULAR RIGHT POSTERIOR teeth.				
4. Demonstrate the USE of the mirror and explorer for calculus detection on the LINGUAL aspect of the MANDIBULAR RIGHT POSTERIOR teeth.				

Instructor _____

Performance Check Time _____

Comments: _____

_____

_____

_____

MANDIBULAR ANTERIOR TEETH (#27–#22)

LINGUAL ASPECT

Instrumentation of the lingual surfaces of the mandibular teeth may be accomplished with the operator positioned at the side or in back of the patient. Since either position is acceptable, instructions will be given for both situations. You may notice that you prefer the side position for the surfaces toward you and the back position for the surfaces away from you. Both positions are often utilized for this area. Practice both positions and develop a system that is most comfortable for you.

SIDE POSITION

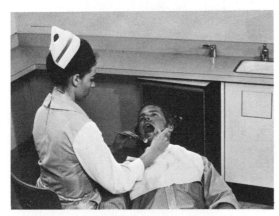

1. Position yourself at the side of the patient.

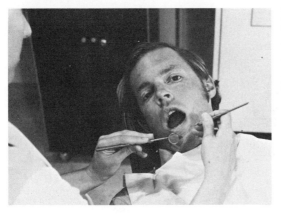

2. Direct the patient to turn his head toward you. If he is not in a supine position, ask him to lower his chin so that the occlusal plane of the mandibular teeth is parallel to the floor. This is especially helpful if you are using direct vision.

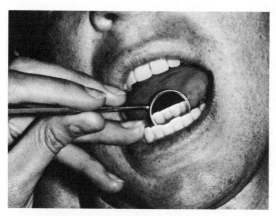

3. You may use direct or indirect vision for this area with the mirror retracting the tongue and reflecting the light. Your mirror finger rest is first established on the occlusal of the mandibular right bicuspid and should move to the lateral incisor as you progress.

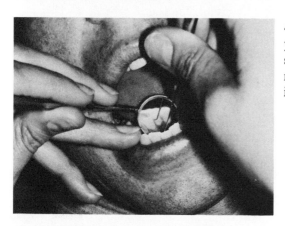

4. Pick up the explorer and establish your instrument finger rest on the incisal surfaces. Keep your finger rest to the right of the area on which you are working.

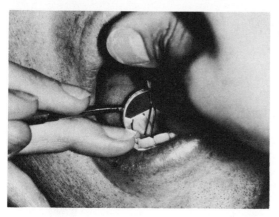

5. Begin exploring the distal surface of the mandibular right cuspid.

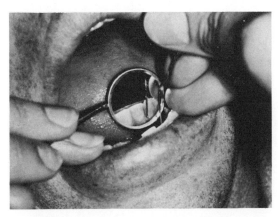

6. Continue exploring the surfaces toward you, up to and including the mesial surface of the mandibular left cuspid. Move your mirror and instrument finger rests along as you go from the right to the left cuspid.

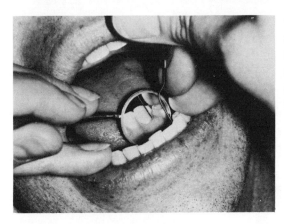

7. When you have finished exploring all of the surfaces toward you, then explore the surfaces away from you, beginning with the distal surface of the left cuspid. Keep your finger rest to the right of the area you are instrumenting.

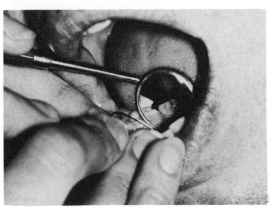

8. Continue exploring the surfaces away from you, up to and including the mesial surfaces of the right cuspid. Remember to keep moving the mirror and finger rests as you work from the left to the right cuspid.

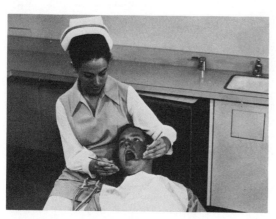

BACK POSITION

1. Position yourself in back of the patient.

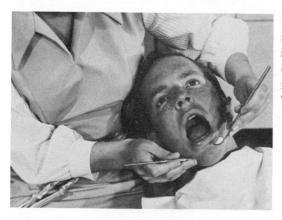

2. Direct the patient to turn his head slightly to the right. If he is not in the supine position, direct him to lower his chin so that the occlusal plane of the mandibular teeth is parallel to the floor. This will facilitate direct vision.

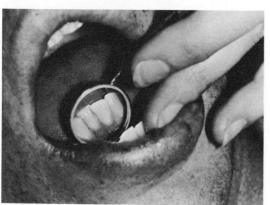

3. You may use either direct or indirect vision in this area, with the mirror retracting the tongue and reflecting light. You will usually use direct vision exclusively when working from a back position. Reach around the patient's head to establish one of the two possible mirror finger rests:

a. Establish your finger rest on the labial surface of the mandibular left cuspid.

or

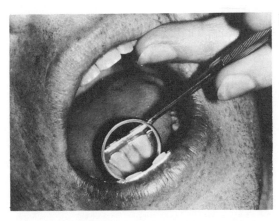

b. Establish your finger rest on the incisal surface of the maxillary cuspid.

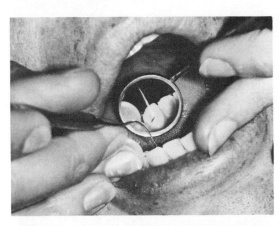

4. **Pick up the** explorer and establish a **finger rest on** the incisal or occlusal sur**faces of adjacent** teeth to the right of the **working area.**

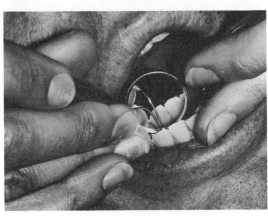

5. Begin exploring the distal surface of the mandibular right cuspid.

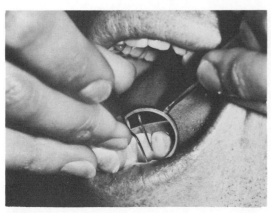

6. Continue exploring the surfaces toward you, including the mesial surface of the left cuspid. Move your mirror and finger rests along as you go from the right to the left side of the mouth.

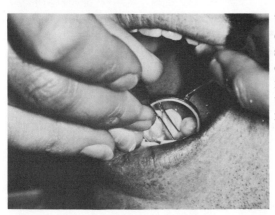

7. When you reach the left cuspid, begin exploring the surfaces away from you, starting with the distal surface of the left cuspid. Keep shifting your instrument finger rest as you go along and adjust the mirror so that you are constantly reflecting light on the working area.

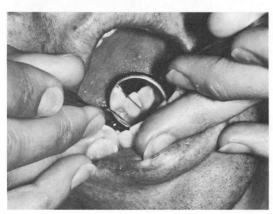

8. Continue exploring the surfaces away from you until you reach the mesial surface of the right cuspid.

MANDIBULAR ANTERIOR TEETH (#27-#22)

LABIAL ASPECT

Instrumentation on the labial surfaces of the mandibular anterior teeth may be accomplished with the operator positioned at the side or in back of the patient. Since either position is acceptable, instructions will be given for both situations. The entire procedure is first described for the side position.

As you practice both positions, you may notice that you prefer the side position for the surfaces toward you and the back position for the surfaces away from you. Combinations of the two positions are often utilized on the maxillary and mandibular anterior teeth. It is best to practice and develop a system that is most comfortable for you.

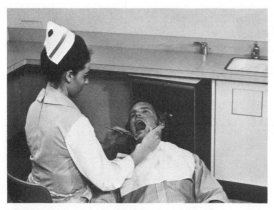

1. Position yourself at the side of the patient.

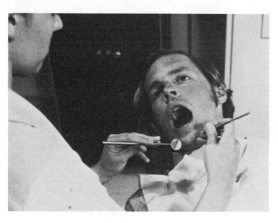

2. Direct the patient to turn his head toward you.

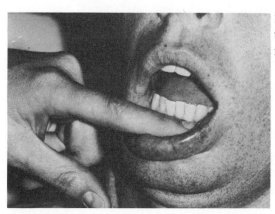

3. You do not need to use the mirror for this area. Use your left index finger to retract the lower lip and use direct vision.

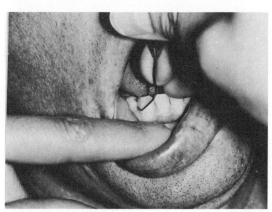

4. Pick up the explorer with your right hand and establish one of the two possible instrument finger rests for this area:
a. Place your ring finger on the incisal surfaces of the teeth adjacent to your working area.

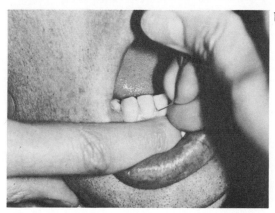

b. Place your left index finger firmly against the attached gingiva in the mandibular anterior area. Then establish your instrument finger rest on your left index finger.

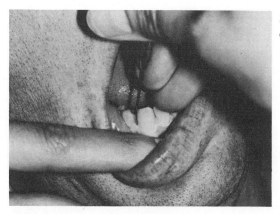

5. Begin by exploring the distal surface of the mandibular right cuspid.

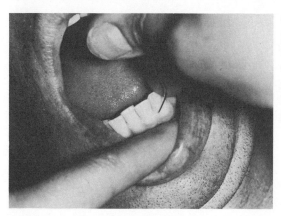

6. Continue exploring all proximal surfaces toward you, up to and including the mesial surfaces of the mandibular left cuspid. Make sure you are moving your finger rest so that it is constantly to the right of the area in which you are working.

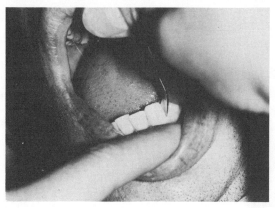

7. When you have finished exploring all of the surfaces toward you, begin to explore all surfaces away from you, beginning with the distal surface of the mandibular left cuspid.

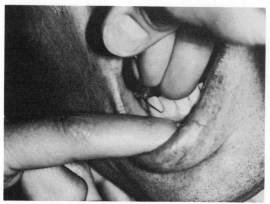

8. Continue exploring the surfaces away from you, up to and including the mesial surface of the mandibular right cuspid. Again, keep moving the finger rest along so that it is just to the right of the area on which you are working.

BACK POSITION

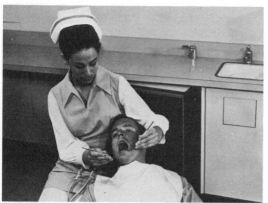

1. Position yourself in back of the patient.

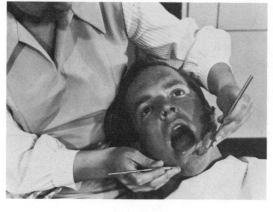

2. Direct the patient to turn his head to the right.

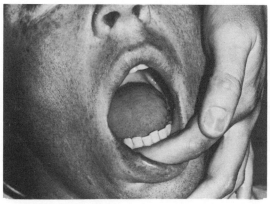

3. You do not need to use the mirror for this area. Retract the lower lip with the left index finger and use direct vision.

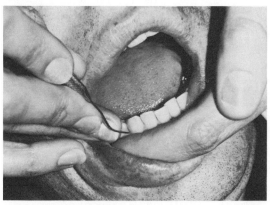

4. Pick up the explorer with your right hand and establish a finger rest on the incisal surfaces to the right of the area to be explored. Begin by exploring the distal surface of the mandibular right cuspid.

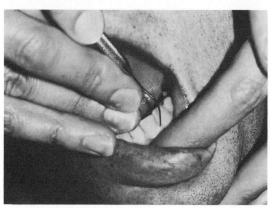

5. Continue exploring all the surfaces toward you, up to and including the mesial surface of the mandibular left cuspid. Make sure that you are moving your finger rest so that it is to the right of the area on which you are working.

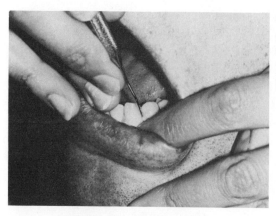

6. When you have finished exploring all of the surfaces facing towards you, begin to explore all of the surfaces facing away from you, beginning with the distal surface of the mandibular left cuspid.

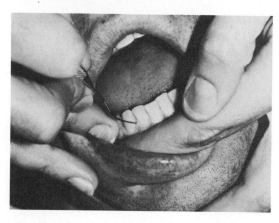

7. Continue exploring the surfaces away from you, up to and including the mesial surface of the mandibular right cuspid. Remember to keep moving your finger rest so that it is always to the right of your working area.

Performance Checklist for Lesson A: Detecting Calculus with the Mirror and Explorer

Name _____

School _____

Date _____

NOTE: The instructor may designate specific operator positioning for this performance check OR the student may be allowed to utilize the position or combination of positions which she prefers.

		#1		#2	
		SATISFACTORY	UNSATISFACTORY	SATISFACTORY	UNSATISFACTORY
5.	Demonstrate the appropriate FULCRUM for the explorer on the LABIAL aspect of the MANDIBULAR ANTERIOR teeth.				
6.	Demonstrate the USE of the explorer for calculus detection on the LABIAL aspect of the MANDIBULAR ANTERIOR teeth.				
7.	Demonstrate the appropriate FULCRUMS for the mirror and explorer on the LINGUAL aspect of the MANDIBULAR ANTERIOR teeth.				
8.	Demonstrate the USE of the mirror and explorer for calculus detection on the LINGUAL aspect of the MANDIBULAR ANTERIOR teeth.				

Instructor _____

Performance Check Time _____

Comments: _____

_____

_____

MANDIBULAR LEFT POSTERIOR TEETH (#21–#17)

Buccal Aspect

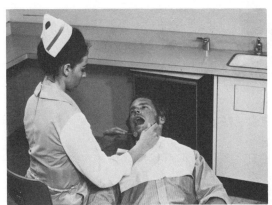

1. Position yourself at the side of the patient.

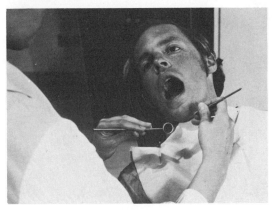

2. Tell the patient to turn his head toward you.

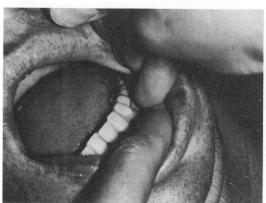

3. Use direct vision in this area if possible. Use the mirror to retract the buccal mucosa and reflect light on the working area. You may need to use indirect vision to see the distal surfaces of the molars. Your mirror finger rest is on the labial surface of the maxillary left cuspid.

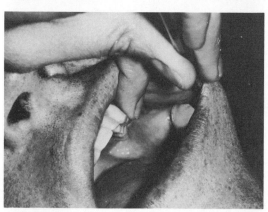

4. You may establish your instrument finger rest by:

a. Placing your ring finger on the bucco-occlusal surfaces of the teeth adjacent to the working area.

and

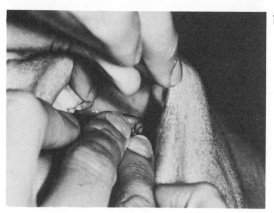

b. Placing the left index finger firmly against the attached gingiva in the mandibular left posterior area. Then establishing your finger rest on the left index finger.

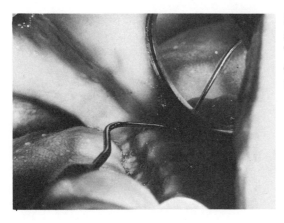

5. Begin exploring the buccal and mesial surfaces of the posterior-most molar. Then explore the distal surface and proceed to the next tooth. Continue forward to the first bicuspid.

MANDIBULAR LEFT POSTERIOR TEETH (#21–#17)

LINGUAL ASPECT

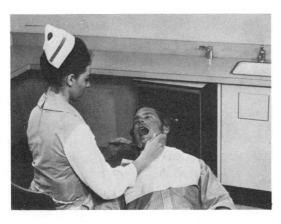

1. Position yourself at the side of the patient.

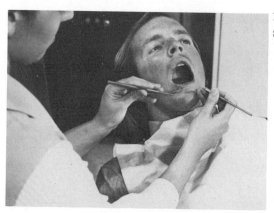

2. Direct the patient to turn his head slightly away from you.

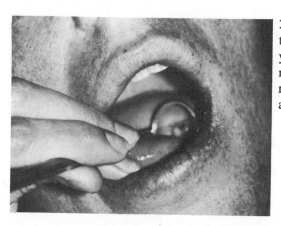

3. Use direct vision with the mirror retracting the tongue and reflecting light on your working area. Your mirror finger rest is on the occlusal surfaces of the mandibular right bicuspid to the lateral area.

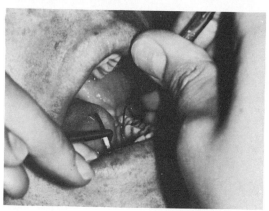

4. Establish your instrument finger rest on the buccal and occlusal surfaces of the teeth adjacent to your working area. Begin exploring the lingual and mesial surfaces of the posterior-most molar. Then explore the distal surface and proceed with the next tooth. Continue forward to the first bicuspid.

Performance Checklist for Lesson A: Detecting Calculus with the Mirror and Explorer

Name _____

School _____

Date _____

	#1		#2	
	SATISFACTORY	UNSATISFACTORY	SATISFACTORY	UNSATISFACTORY
9. Demonstrate the appropriate FULCRUMS for the mirror and explorer on the BUCCAL aspect of the MANDIBULAR LEFT POSTERIOR teeth.				
10. Demonstrate the USE of the mirror and explorer for calculus detection on the BUCCAL aspect of the MANDIBULAR LEFT POSTERIOR teeth.				
11. Demonstrate the appropriate FULCRUMS for the mirror and explorer on the LINGUAL aspect of the MANDIBULAR LEFT POSTERIOR teeth.				
12. Demonstrate the USE of the mirror and explorer for calculus detection on the LINGUAL aspect of the MANDIBULAR LEFT POSTERIOR teeth.				

Instructor _____

Performance Check Time _____

Comments: _____

_____

_____

_____

MAXILLARY RIGHT POSTERIOR TEETH (#1–#5)

BUCCAL ASPECT

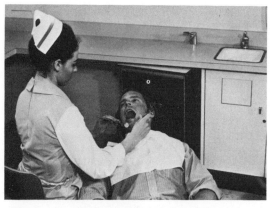

1. Position yourself at the side of the patient. The patient's head should be level with or lower than your elbow.

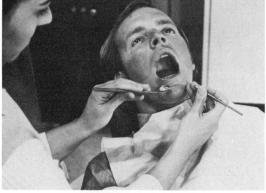

2. Direct the patient to turn his head slightly away from you. This position allows maximum direct vision.

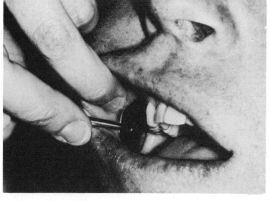

3. Your mirror finger rest may be established by:
a. Placing the ring finger on the buccal mucosa and gently pulling the cheek away from the teeth.

or

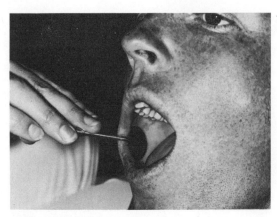

b. Placing the ring finger on the shank of the mirror and gently pulling the cheek away from the teeth.

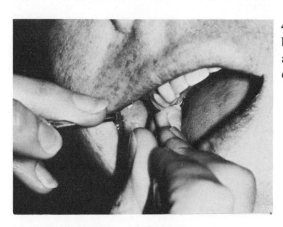

4. Establish your instrument finger rest by placing your ring finger on the buccal and occlusal surfaces of the teeth and closest to your working area.

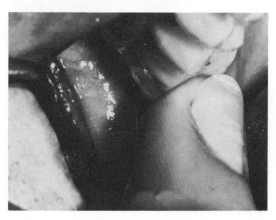

5. Explore the buccal and mesial surfaces of the posterior-most molar. Then explore the distal surface of this tooth and proceed with the next tooth. Continue forward to the first bicuspid. Remember to move your finger rest so that it is always on the teeth closest to your working area.

MAXILLARY RIGHT POSTERIOR TEETH (#1–#5)

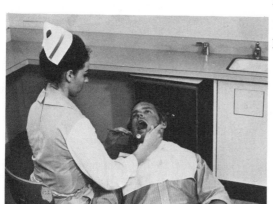

LINGUAL ASPECT

1. Position yourself at the side of the patient.

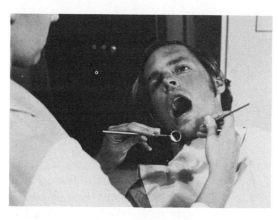

2. Ask the patient to turn his head toward you.

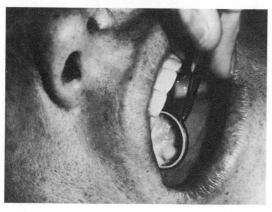

3. You may use direct or indirect vision in this area with the mirror reflecting light. Your mirror finger rest is on the labial surface of the maxillary left cuspid.

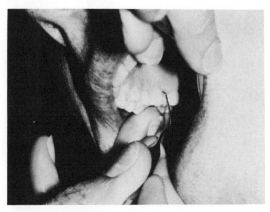

4. Pick up the explorer with your right hand and utilize any of the following instrument finger rests:
a. Place your ring finger on the occlusal surfaces of the adjacent teeth.

or

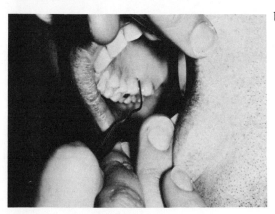

b. Place your ring finger on the labio-incisal surfaces of the mandibular anterior teeth.

or

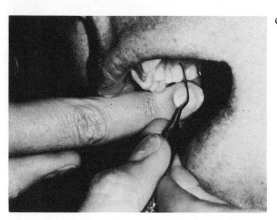

c. Place the index finger of your left hand on the occlusal surfaces of the adjacent teeth. Then place the ring finger of your right hand on the left index finger. Since you cannot use the mirror with this finger rest, you must use direct vision. Begin exploring the lingual and mesial surfaces of the posterior-most molar. Then explore the distal surface and proceed with the next tooth. Continue forward to the first bicuspid.

Performance Checklist for Lesson A: Detecting Calculus with the Mirror and Explorer

Name _____

School _____

Date _____

		#1		#2	
		SATISFACTORY	UNSATISFACTORY	SATISFACTORY	UNSATISFACTORY
13.	Demonstrate the appropriate FULCRUMS for the mirror and explorer on the BUCCAL aspect of the MANDIBULAR RIGHT POSTERIOR teeth.				
14.	Demonstrate the USE of the mirror and explorer for calculus detection on the BUCCAL aspect of the MAXILLARY RIGHT POSTERIOR teeth.				
15.	Demonstrate the appropriate FULCRUMS for the mirror and explorer on the LINGUAL aspect of the MAXILLARY RIGHT POSTERIOR teeth.				
16.	Demonstrate the USE of the mirror and explorer for calculus detection on the LINGUAL aspect of the MAXILLARY RIGHT POSTERIOR teeth.				

Instructor _____

Performance Check Time _____

Comments: _____

_____

_____

_____

MAXILLARY ANTERIOR TEETH (#6–#11)

LABIAL ASPECT

Instrumentation on the labial surfaces of the maxillary anterior teeth may be accomplished from a side or a back position. Either position or a combination of the two is acceptable.

SIDE POSITION

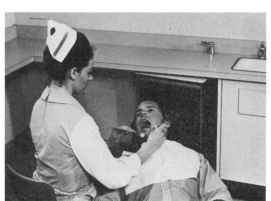

1. Position yourself at the side of the patient.

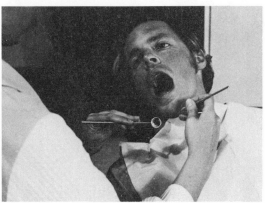

2. Direct the patient to turn his head toward you.

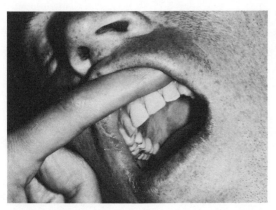

3. You do not need to use the mirror for this area. Retract the upper left lip with the left index finger and use direct vision.

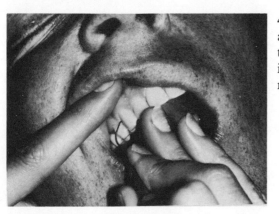

4. Establish a finger rest on the labial and incisal surfaces just to the right of the area to be explored. Begin by exploring the distal surface of the maxillary right cuspid.

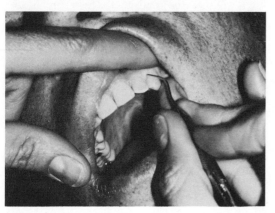

5. Continue exploring all the proximal surfaces toward you, up to and including the mesial surface of the maxillary left cuspid. Make sure that you are moving your finger rest so that it is constantly to the right of the area on which you are working.

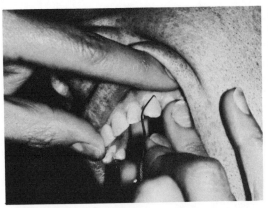

6. When you have finished exploring all of the surfaces facing toward you, begin to explore all the surfaces facing away from you, beginning with the distal surface of the maxillary left cuspid.

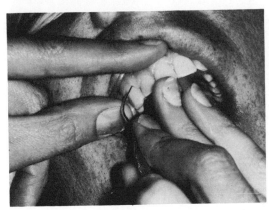

7. Continue exploring the surfaces away from you, up to and including the mesial surface of the maxillary right cuspid. Again, keep moving the finger rest along so that it is just to the right of the area on which you are working.

BACK POSITION

You may wish to explore the surfaces away from you from the back position, as you did on the mandibular anterior teeth.

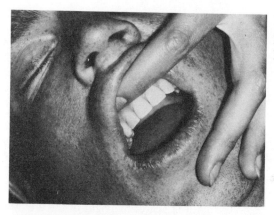

1. Approach the patient from a back position and retract the upper lip with your left index finger.

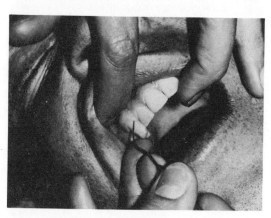

2. Explore the surfaces away from you, beginning with the mesial of the right cuspid.

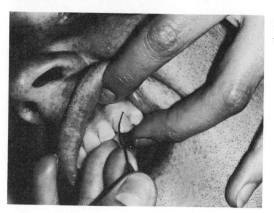

3. Continue exploring up to and including the distal surface of the left cuspid.

MAXILLARY ANTERIOR TEETH (#6–#11)

LINGUAL ASPECT

Instrumentation on the lingual surfaces of the maxillary anterior teeth may also be accomplished from a side or back position. Again, instructions will be given for both situations.

Combinations for the two positions may be utilized for the lingual aspect also.

SIDE POSITION

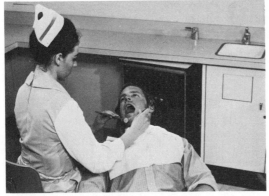

1. Position yourself at the side of the patient.

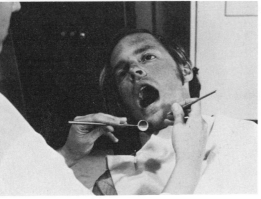

2. Direct the patient to turn his head toward you.

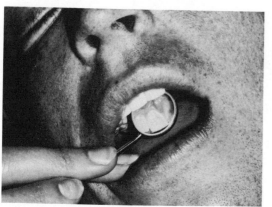

3. You must use the mirror for indirect vision in this area. Establish your finger rest on either of the two possible positions listed below. Adjust your mirror so that you can see the lingual of the right cuspid. Make sure you are also reflecting light on your working area.

a. Place your left ring finger on the occlusal surfaces of the mandibular right bicuspid-cuspid area.

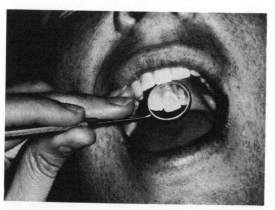

or

b. Place your left ring finger on the buccal surfaces of the maxillary right bicuspids.

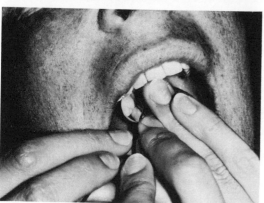

4. Establish an instrument finger rest on the labial and incisal surfaces of the right central and lateral. Begin exploring the surfaces toward you, beginning with the distal surfaces of the right cuspid.

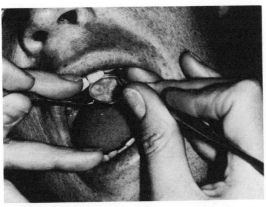

5. Continue exploring the surfaces toward you, up to and including the mesial surface of the left cuspid. Move your finger rest along and keep it to the right of your working area.

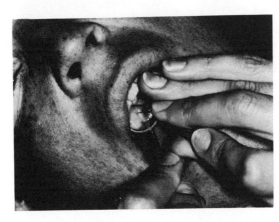

6. Then explore the surfaces away from you, beginning on the distal surface of the left cuspid and ending on the mesial surface of the right cuspid.

BACK POSITION

1. Position yourself in back of the patient.

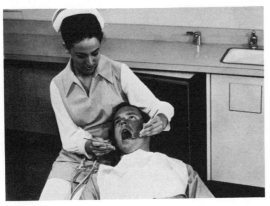

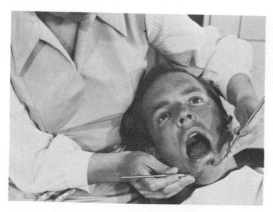

2. Ask the patient to turn his head to the right.

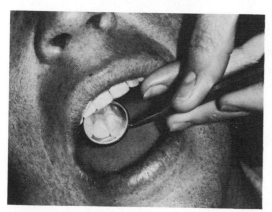

3. You must use the mirror for indirect vision in this area. Reach around the patient's head and establish your finger rest on the incisal surface of the maxillary left cuspid. Adjust your mirror so you can see the lingual of the right cuspid. Make sure that your mirror is also reflecting light on the working area.

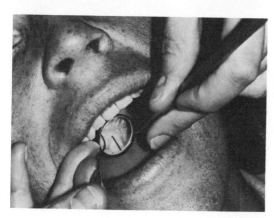

4. Establish an instrument finger rest on the buccal and occlusal surfaces of the maxillary right first bicuspid. Begin exploring the distal surface of the right cuspid.

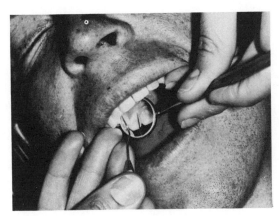

5. When you have reached the left cuspid, begin exploring the surfaces away from you, starting on the distal surface of the left cuspid and ending on the mesial surface of the right cuspid. Don't forget to keep moving your finger rest as you progress from left to right. As you move, your finger rest must always be to the right of your working area.

Performance Checklist for Lesson A: Detecting Calculus with the Mirror and Explorer

Name _____

School _____

Date _____

NOTE: The instructor may designate specific operator positioning for this performance check OR the student may be allowed to utilize the position or combination that she most prefers.

	#1		#2	
	SATISFACTORY	UNSATISFACTORY	SATISFACTORY	UNSATISFACTORY
17. Demonstrate the appropriate FULCRUM for the explorer on the LABIAL aspect of the MAXILLARY ANTERIOR teeth.				
18. Demonstrate the USE of the explorer for calculus detection on the LABIAL aspect of the MAXILLARY ANTERIOR teeth.				
19. Demonstrate the appropriate FULCRUMS for the mirror and explorer on the LINGUAL aspect of the MAXILLARY ANTERIOR teeth.				
20. Demonstrate the USE of the mirror and explorer for calculus detection on the LINGUAL aspect of the MAXILLARY ANTERIOR teeth.				

Instructor _____

Performance Check Time _____

Comments: _____

_____

_____

MAXILLARY LEFT POSTERIOR TEETH (#12–#16)

BUCCAL ASPECT

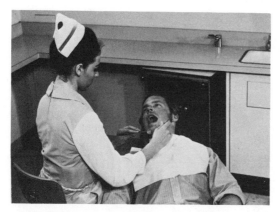

1. Position yourself at the side of the patient.

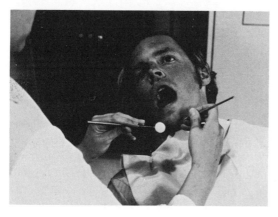

2. Direct the patient to turn his head toward you.

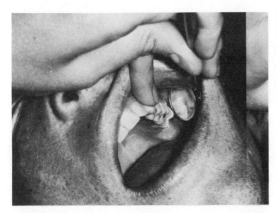

3. Establish your mirror finger rest on the buccal of the maxillary left cuspid area. Use your mirror to retract the buccal mucosa. You should be able to use direct vision in this area—except for the posterior-most molars.

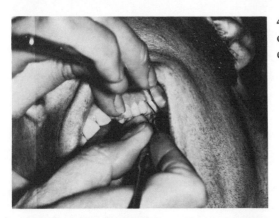

4. Establish your instrument finger rest on the occlusal surfaces of the teeth closest to your working area.

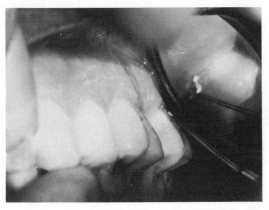

5. Explore the buccal and mesial surfaces of the posterior-most molar. Then explore the distal surface of this tooth. Move on to the buccal and mesial surfaces and then the distal surface of the next tooth. Continue exploring each tooth in this manner, from the last tooth in the quadrant to the first bicuspid.

MAXILLARY LEFT POSTERIOR TEETH (#12–#16)

LINGUAL ASPECT

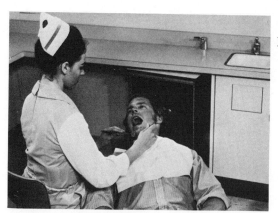

1. Position yourself at the side of the patient.

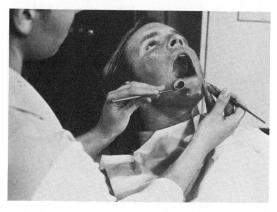

2. Direct the patient to raise his head and turn it slightly away from you.

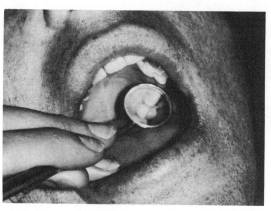

3. Use direct vision if possible, but always use the mirror to reflect light on your working area. Your mirror finger rest may be established by:

a. Placing the ring finger on the occlusal surfaces of the mandibular right cuspid-bicuspid area.

or

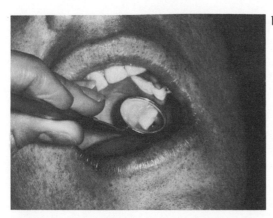

b. Placing the ring finger on the buccal surfaces of the maxillary right cuspid-bicuspid area.

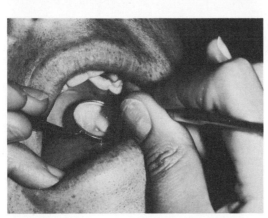

4. There are two possible instrument finger rests for this area:

a. Placing the ring finger on the buccal and occlusal surfaces of the teeth adjacent to your working area.

or

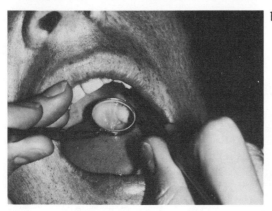

b. Placing your ring finger on the incisal surfaces of the mandibular left cuspid and lateral incisors.

Begin exploring the lingual and mesial surfaces of the posterior-most molar. Then explore the distal surface and proceed with the next tooth. Continue forward to the first bicuspid.

Performance Checklist for Lesson A: Detecting Calculus with the Mirror and Explorer

Name _____

School _____

Date _____

	#1		#2	
	SATISFACTORY	UNSATISFACTORY	SATISFACTORY	UNSATISFACTORY
21. Demonstrate the appropriate FULCRUMS for the mirror and explorer on the BUCCAL aspect of the MAXILLARY LEFT POSTERIOR teeth.				
22. Demonstrate the USE of the mirror and explorer for calculus detection on the BUCCAL aspect of the MAXILLARY LEFT POSTERIOR teeth.				
23. Demonstrate the appropriate FULCRUMS for the mirror and explorer on the LINGUAL aspect of the MAXILLARY LEFT POSTERIOR teeth.				
24. Demonstrate the USE of the mirror and explorer for calculus detection on the LINGUAL aspect of the MAXILLARY LEFT POSTERIOR teeth.				

Instructor _____

Performance Check Time _____

Comments: _____

_____

_____

_____

Review Questions for Lesson A: Detecting Calculus with the Mirror and Explorer

Circle the letter of the *one* best answer.

Read the following phrases before answering questions 1 and 2.

    1. detection of supragingival calculus
    2. detection of subgingival calculus
    3. indirect vision
    4. retraction of cheeks, lips, and tongue
    5. determination of root smoothness
    6. illumination
    7. determination of completion of prophylaxis

1. Which of the above phrases best describe the uses of the mirror?
    a. 1, 3, 4, 6, 7
    b. 1, 3, 5, 6, 7
    c. 2, 3, 4, 5, 6
    d. 2, 4, 5, 6

2. Which of the above phrases best describe the uses of the explorer?
    a. 2, 3, 6, 7
    b. 1, 4, 6, 7
    c. 3, 5, 6, 7
    d. 1, 2, 5, 7

3. The very end of the explorer is referred to as the:
    a. tip
    b. point
    c. end
    d. toe
    e. blade

4. The terminal 1 to 2 mm of the working end of the explorer is called the:
    a. tip
    b. point
    c. end
    d. toe
    e. blade

5. The explorer may be designed:
    a. as a single-ended instrument
    b. as a double-ended instrument
    c. with paired working ends
    d. with dissimilar working ends
    e. all of the above

Read the following descriptive phrases before answering questions 6 and 7:

    1. used primarily for calculus detection
    2. used primarily for caries detection
    3. excellent for deep pockets and furcations
    4. too thick for good tactile sensitivity
    5. easily adapted to all tooth surfaces

6. Which of the above phrases best describe the #17 explorer?
    a. 1, 3, 4
    b. 1, 3, 5
    c. 2, 3, 5
    d. 2, 3, 4
    e. 2, 4, 5

7. Which of the above phrases best describe the shepherd's hook explorer?
    a. 1, 3, 5
    b. 2, 3, 5
    c. 2, 4
    d. 1, 4
    e. 2, 5

8. The explorer should be used:
    a. prior to scaling
    b. during gross scaling
    c. during definitive scaling
    d. after root planing
    e. a and d only
    f. all of the above

To correct your replies, turn to the Answer Key on page 159.

Lesson B: *Detecting Periodontal Pockets with the Periodontal Probe*

Selection of calculus & Periodontal Pockets

The *periodontal probe* is an instrument that is used for examining periodontal pockets. With its calibrated working end, the probe enables the operator to approximate the depth, topography, and character of the periodontal pocket.

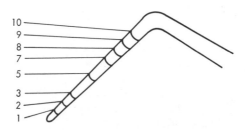

Probes vary in cross-sectional design and millimeter markings. They may be rectangular (flat), oval, or round in cross section, but all are relatively slender to allow easy insertion into the sulcus or pocket. The calibrated working end is marked in millimeters at varying intervals to facilitate reading of pocket depth measurements. The most commonly used probes are marked at 1, 2, 3, and then 5, 7, 8, 9, and 10 mm as shown in the drawing above. Some probes are marked at every millimeter up to 10, but these are not recommended because they are very difficult to read when placed subgingivally. Pocket measurements are recorded preoperatively and postoperatively whether the procedure is surgical or prophylactic. Comparison of these measurements is an adjunct to the evaluation of tissue response.

Periodontal measurements are taken by gently inserting the probe under the marginal gingiva and moving it down to the epithelial attachment. You may find that passage of your probe to the epithelial attachment is obstructed by calculus. If so, you will feel your probe encountering a hard, unyielding ledge. Lift the probe gently away from the tooth against the tissue wall of the pocket and attempt to proceed vertically again, bypassing the obstruction. When the obstruction is calculus, the probe will move deeper into the pocket. Eventually your progress will be impeded by another obstruction that feels relatively soft, elastic, and resilient. This you should recognize as the epithelial attachment—the point from which your reading should be taken. The probe should always be kept as nearly parallel to the long axis of the tooth as possible to insure correct measurement. Tilting the probe sideways or away from the tooth will result in an inaccurate reading. Also be sure to keep the working end well-adapted to the tooth surface, or you may puncture the epithelium as illustrated below:

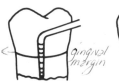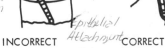

| CORRECT (Probe is parallel with long axis of tooth) | INCORRECT (Probe is not parallel with long axis of tooth) | CORRECT (Probe is well-adapted) | INCORRECT (Probe is not well-adapted) |

Six periodontal measurements are taken on each tooth: three from the buccal (disto-buccal, buccal, and mesio-buccal), and three from the lingual (disto-lingual, lingual, and mesio-lingual). Measurements are taken from the base of the pocket or epithelial attachment to the margin of the free gingiva. As you probe, you will be instructed to keep the probe within the sulcus and gently "bob" up and down off the epithelial attachment. While you will routinely record only six measurements per tooth, this bobbing technique allows detection of insidious pockets between the normal recording areas.

The following exercise will teach you to take these six specific measurements on a molar and an anterior tooth. If you are working on a patient, you will be able to measure the actual depth of the sulcus. If you are working on a manikin, which unfortunately lacks epithelial attachments, you will have to use your imagination and concentrate on inserting the probe to different depths and reading the markings.

Position your patient, wash your hands, and begin working on the mandibular right first molar.

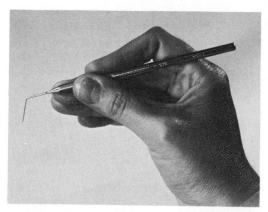

1. Grasp the periodontal probe with a modified pen grasp.
If you are working on a patient, retract the buccal mucosa with the mirror.

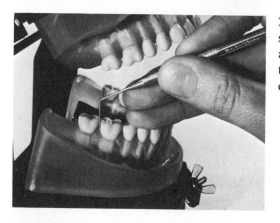

2. Establish a finger rest on the occlusal surfaces of the mandibular right bicuspids and place the tip of the probe just above the free margin of the gingiva in the area of the distal line angle.

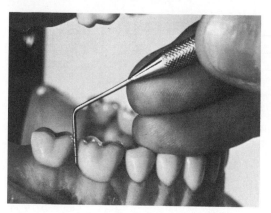

3. Now move the probe as close to the contact area as possible and keep it parallel to the long axis of the tooth. Gently insert the tip under the free margin and carefully slide down to the epithelial attachment. When you are sure that you feel the resistance of the attachment, read the measurement for the disto-buccal area.

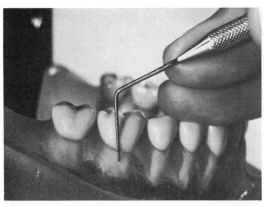

4. *Keep the tip in the sulcus and gently "bob" the tip up and down slightly* as you move around the line angle toward the buccal surface. Remember to keep the probe well-adapted and parallel to the tooth surface. Now read the measurement for the buccal area. The picture shows a hypothetical 2 mm measurement. Note, however, that in this picture the probe is not parallel to the long axis of the tooth. The same pocket, recorded with correct adaptation of the probe, will actually read less than 2 mm.

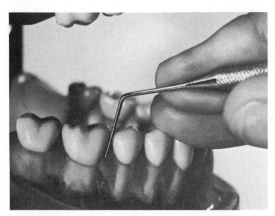

5. Continue moving the tip up and down in the sulcus until you are as far into the mesial contact as possible and read the measurement for the mesio-buccal area. The "bobbing" action allows you to follow the epithelial attachment around the tooth and is important in determining the topography as well as the depth of the pocket.

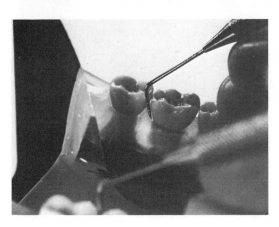

6. Using the same finger rest, begin probing on the lingual surface. Measure the depth in the disto-lingual area and use the mirror for indirect vision if necessary. The hypothetical measurement in the picture is approximately 7 mm.

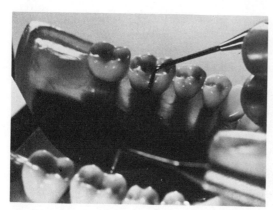

7. Probe around the line angle and measure the lingual area.

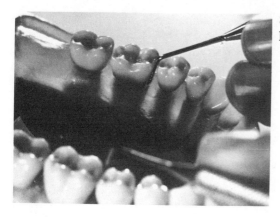

8. Now measure the depth in the mesiolingual area.

After you have learned to use the probe on a posterior tooth, proceed to practice on an anterior tooth. The six measurements are the same, but are taken much closer together because the tooth is smaller. Begin working on the labial aspect of any mandibular anterior tooth.

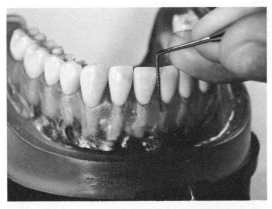

1. Establish a finger rest on the incisal surfaces of the adjacent teeth and insert the probe in the mesio-labial area.

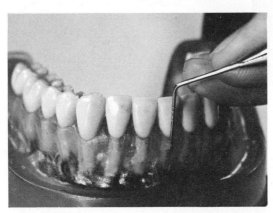

2. Gently move the probe into position on the labial surface and read the measurement.

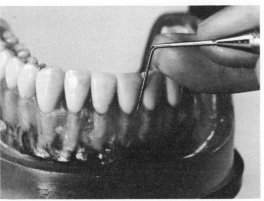

3. Measure the disto-labial depth. Be sure to move the probe very gently on the anterior teeth because the tissue is usually very tight in this area. Even when there is a deep narrow pocket, the gingiva around the neck of an anterior tooth may be so firm that it will be difficult to insert the probe.

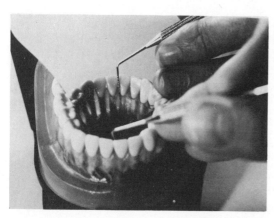

4. Now use your mirror for illumination and indirect vision as you probe the disto-lingual area.

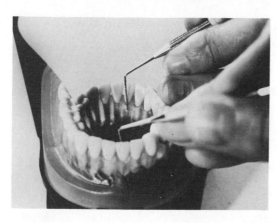

5. Measure the depth in the lingual area.

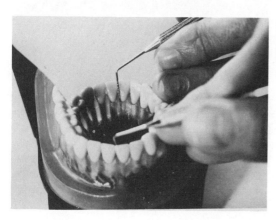

6. Measure the mesio-lingual depth, making sure that the probe is parallel to the long axis of the tooth and as far into the interproximal area as possible.

Periodontal measurements are usually taken first from the buccal aspect and then from the lingual. Practice using your probe on at least one quadrant of the mouth in this manner. Measure the disto-buccal, buccal, and mieso-buccal depths of the posterior-most molar in the quadrant and then take these same measurements on the next tooth. After you have reached the central incisor, begin measuring the lingual depths on that tooth and continue probing until you have measured all of the lingual areas on the posterior-most molar. If you are probing the entire mouth, measure the facial surfaces of the maxillary and mandibular arch, and then measure the lingual surfaces of both arches.

Review Questions for Lesson B: Detecting Periodontal Pockets with the Periodontal Probe

1. The most common markings on the periodontal probe are at:
   a. 1, 2, 4, 6, 8, 9 and 10 mm
   b. 1, 2, 3, 4, 6, 8, 9, and 10 mm
   c. 1, 2, 3, 5, 7, 8, 9, and 10 mm
   d. 1, 2, 5, 7, 8, 9, and 10 mm
   e. every millimeter up to 10 mm

2. Periodontal measurements are taken from the:
   a. epithelial attachment to the occlusal surface
   b. epithelial attachment to the CEJ
   c. CEJ to the free gingival margin
   d. epithelial attachment to the free gingival margin
   e. b and d

3. If you meet resistance after inserting the periodontal probe into the sulcus, you should:
   a. remove the probe and select one with a narrow diameter
   b. force the probe beyond the obstruction
   c. remove the probe and reinsert it in a different spot
   d. lift the probe away from the tooth and attempt to move apically
   e. read the probe and record the measurement

4. How should the periodontal probe be inserted into the sulcus?
   a. parallel to the long axis of the tooth
   b. perpendicular to the long axis of the tooth
   c. very gently with a palm grasp
   d. with a short, oblique stroke
   e. with a horizontal "bobbing" motion

5. The sulcular epithelium is likely to be punctured by the point if the probe is:
   a. parallel to the long axis of the tooth
   b. not parallel to the long axis of the tooth
   c. well adapted to the tooth
   d. not well adapted to the tooth
   e. inserted vertically

To correct your replies, turn to the Answer Key on page 159.

Performance Checklist for Lesson B: Detecting Periodontal Pockets with the Periodontal Probe

Name _____

School _____

Date _____

		#1		#2	
		SATISFACTORY	UNSATISFACTORY	SATISFACTORY	UNSATISFACTORY
25.	Demonstrate the use of the periodontal probe to measure six specific areas on any molar.				
26.	Demonstrate the use of the periodontal probe to measure six specific areas on an anterior tooth.				

Instructor _____

Performance Check Time _____

Comments: _____

_____

_____

_____

Lesson C: *Using Compressed Air*

Compressed air can be a very useful adjunct to your dental hygiene armamentarium. It is used in detecting supragingival calculus, deflecting tissue
to view subgingival calculus, and clearing the field of operation of saliva.
Calculus that is wet with saliva can be difficult to detect, especially in the
final stages of the prophylaxis or when only light supragingival calculus is
present. Thorough drying of the calculus with a steady stream of air will
make the calculus appear chalk-like so that it can be distinguished easily
from tooth structure. Also, dried calculus is easier to detect with the explorer because there is less chance of slipping over it. It may be necessary
that you dry the teeth several times before you can be sure that all supragingival calculus has been removed. Dry the teeth well and examine them
for residual calculus very carefully with your mirror and explorer. Rescale
the teeth as necessary, and then dry and examine them again.

When checking for the presence of subgingival calculus, you may use
compressed air to deflect tissue, allowing a more thorough examination of
the subgingival area. When a strong, steady stream of air is directed into the
gingival sulcus, the free gingiva will be deflected, making the sulcus visible.
If there is calculus in the area, you will be able to see the dark brown to
black deposits on the root surface.

There are certain precautions that should be taken when using compressed air. A stream of air can cause discomfort to a patient with deep
caries or hypersensitive teeth. If air is used at all, short jets of warm air
may sometimes be tolerated by the patient; however, when sensitivity is too
great, a saliva ejector should be used and the teeth dried with a gauze
square instead. This method is a less effective but more comfortable alter-
native.

USE OF AIR FOR CALCULUS DETECTION

This exercise must be performed on a fellow-student patient. You will need a sterile mirror, an explorer, and an air syringe. Position your patient, wash your hands, and begin working on the mandibular anterior area.

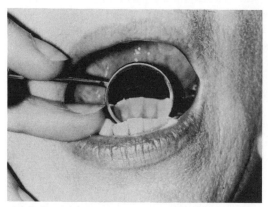

1. Retract the tongue with the mirror. Use the mirror at all times for illumination of the working area and for indirect vision when necessary.

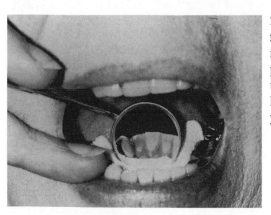

2. If a saliva ejector is not being used, fold a gauze square twice in the same direction and place it in the floor of the patient's mouth under his tongue. Rest the mirror on top of the gauze. This will keep saliva from pooling in the area as you dry the teeth with air.

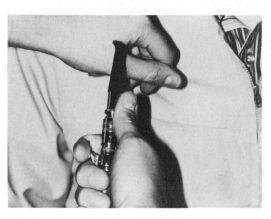

3. Grasp the air syringe with a palm grasp and first test the air flow on your left hand. Make sure that you can control the air to permit a strong steady stream of air to flow from the syringe.

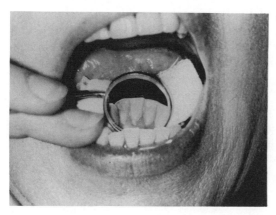

4. Now begin drying the lingual surfaces of the mandibular anterior teeth. Continue blowing a steady stream of air until the teeth are *completely* dry.

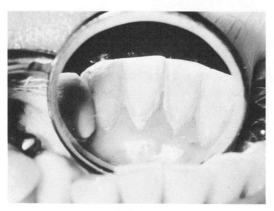

5. Inspect the lingual surfaces carefully by direct and indirect vision. Use your mirror to reflect light onto the area. *Dry supragingival calculus will appear white and chalky.* If the calculus appears to be yellow, it is probably not completely dry yet. You should also use your mirror to transilluminate. When transilluminated, the calculus will appear as a dark shadow on the surface of the tooth.

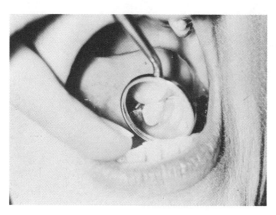

6. Turn your mirror head from side to side as you scan the lingual surfaces so you can see the interproximal areas.

If you have been successful in drying and detecting supragingival calculus in your patient's mouth, use your explorer to feel it (in addition to examining it with the mirror). This basic procedure may be utilized in any area of the mouth where you wish to check for supragingival calculus before, during, or after scaling. The most common areas in which supragingival calculus is found are the lingual surfaces of the mandibular anterior teeth and the buccal surfaces of the maxillary molars. This is true because the ducts of the major salivary glands are located near these teeth, and the abundant flow of saliva in the area provides the calcium for the calcification of bacterial plaque.

USE OF AIR FOR DEFLECTION OF TISSUE

In addition to drying supragingival calculus, you should also practice blowing compressed air into the gingival sulcus. Choose an area such as the buccal surface of the mandibular first molar or cuspid and direct a steady stream of air into the sulcus while holding the air syringe very close to the free margin. Although you will probably not be able to see subgingival calculus on your fellow-student patient, you should be able to see the free gingiva being deflected away from the tooth.

Review Questions for Lesson C: Using Compressed Air

1. Thoroughly dried supragingival calculus appears:
    a. translucent
    b. no different than wet calculus
    c. dark brown to black
    d. chalk-like
    e. smooth and yellow

2. If your patient has hypersensitive teeth or caries, you should use:
    a. a steady, soft stream of air
    b. a soft stream of hot air
    c. short jets of warm air
    d. short jets of cool air
    e. one short blast of air

3. Air is used to deflect the free gingival margin in order to detect:
    a. supragingival calculus
    b. subgingival calculus
    c. the CEJ
    d. smooth root surfaces
    e. inflammation

4. The air syringe is held with a:
    a. modified palm grasp
    b. pen grasp

    c. modified pen grasp

    d. three-finger grasp

    e. palm grasp

5. Dried calculus is easier to detect than wet calculus with the explorer because it is:

    a. harder

    b. softer

    c. less slippery

    d. smoother

    e. darker

To correct your replies, turn to the Answer Key on page 159.

Performance Checklist for Lesson C: Using Compressed Air

Name _____

School _____

Date _____

		#1		#2	
		SATISFACTORY	UNSATISFACTORY	SATISFACTORY	UNSATISFACTORY
27.	Demonstrate the use of compressed air on the lingual aspect of the mandibular anterior teeth to detect supragingival calculus on a fellow-student patient.				
28.	Demonstrate the use of compressed air to deflect the gingiva on a fellow-student patient.				

Instructor _____

Performance Check Time _____

Comments: _____

_____

_____

_____

Lesson D: *Detecting Calculus on Radiographs*

The importance of radiographs in conjunction with prophylaxis technique cannot be overstressed. You should never begin working on a patient without first having viewed the most current radiographs in his chart. Because the clinical appearance of periodontal disease can be very deceiving, radiographs are an invaluable adjunct in determining the height and contour of the alveolar bone as well as in revealing the location of large deposits of subgingival calculus.

Calculus appears *radiopaque* in radiographs. Heavy interproximal calculus will look like a "spur" or a lump. Heavy supragingival calculus is often seen as a "cloud" surrounding the clinical crown of the tooth and is especially noticeable on lower anteriors. Buccal and lingual supragingival or subgingival calculus may appear as a crescent or irregular line near the cervical area of the tooth. It is important to note that only moderate to heavy deposits are evident on radiographs. Lack of evidence of calculus does not mean that subgingival calculus is not present. It does indicate that you will have to rely solely on your explorer to find subgingival calculus. Remember that your explorer is your most important calculus detection instrument and that all other aids should be used only as adjuncts of the explorer.

Although radiographs do not reveal exact bony contours, they do provide some insight into the underlying structure of the periodontium. Bone resorption appears *radiolucent,* but remember that bacterial invasion and inflammation can proceed far into the bone before the bone's calcified structure is sufficiently affected to appear radiolucent. Keep in mind that an X-ray is a two-dimensional representation of a three-dimensional object. Consequently, overlapping of structures will occur. Deficiencies in the radiographic technique must be eliminated because they can be deceiving and will only add to the examiner's problems of interpreting radiographic images. Despite this disadvantage, however, radiographs are vital aids to thorough scaling.

The following radiographs reveal heavy calculus and bone resorption. Examine them carefully and then ask your instructor for a full mouth set of radiographs that you can study. When you think you have detected all of the calculus evident in the radiographs, you should request a performance check.

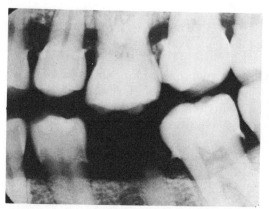

1. This bite-wing radiograph shows heavy calculus spurs on all of the posterior teeth. Notice that the interproximal space between the maxillary first and second molars is almost totally bridged by calculus. Generalized bone loss is also evident.

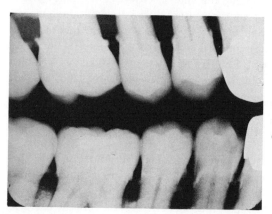

2. Heavy buccal and lingual calculi appear as radiopaque lines across the cervical areas of these mandibular bicuspid teeth. Interproximal spurs and bone loss are also present. Notice the severe vertical bone loss related to the abundant calculus on the mesial surface of the mandibular second bicuspid.

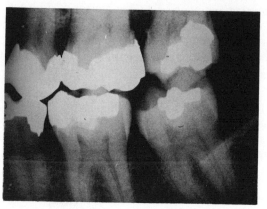

3. The small lumps on these mandibular molars reveal moderate calculus, while the larger spurs on the maxillary molars indicate heavier deposits.

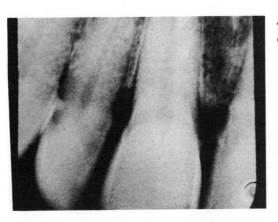

4. There is heavy interproximal calculus on all of these maxillary anterior teeth.

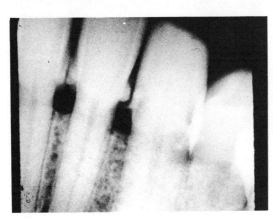

5. These mandibular anterior teeth are heavily encrusted with interproximal calculus. Clinical examination would probably reveal heavy supragingival calculus on the lingual surfaces as well.

Review Questions for Lesson D: Detecting Calculus on Radiographs

1. Interproximal subgingival calculus appears as _____ on radiographs.
      a. radiopaque spurs or lumps
      b. radiolucent spurs or lumps
      c. irregular lines
      d. "clouds"
      e. radiopaque squares

2. Subgingival or supragingival calculus on buccal and lingual surfaces appears as _____ on radiographs.

      a. radiopaque spurs or lumps
      b. radiopaque crescents or irregular lines
      c. radiolucent crescents or irregular lines
      d. radiolucent "clouds"
      e. radiopaque "clouds"

3. Radiographs cannot be used to:
    a. detect heavy interproximal calculus
    b. differentiate between buccal and lingual calculus
    c. detect supragingival calculus
    d. detect bone loss
    e. b and c

4. Radiographs are a useful adjunct to the explorer in the detection of:
    a. smooth sheets of subgingival calculus
    b. light to moderate calculus
    c. the texture of calculus
    d. moderate to heavy calculus
    e. residual fine calculus

To correct your replies, turn to the Answer Key on page 159.

Performance Checklist for Lesson D: Detecting Calculus on Radiographs

Name _____

School _____

Date _____

	#1		#2	
	SATISFACTORY	UNSATISFACTORY	SATISFACTORY	UNSATISFACTORY
29. Examine a full mouth set of radiographs and detect all evident calculus.				

Instructor _____

Performance Check Time _____

Comments: _____

_____

_____

_____

ANSWER KEY

LESSON A

1. a
2. d
3. b
4. a
5. e
6. b
7. c
8. f

LESSON B

1. c
2. d
3. d

4. a
5. d

LESSON C

1. d
2. c
3. b
4. e
5. c

LESSON D

1. a
2. b
3. b
4. d

READING ASSIGNMENTS FOR REVIEW *

A. *Sterilization, Disinfection, and Sanitization:*

Steele, *Dimensions of Dental Hygiene,* pp. 146–153.
Wilkins, *Clinical Practice of the Dental Hygienist,* pp. 15–21; 23–33.

B. *Introduction to Periodontics:*

Glickman, *Clinical Periodontology,* pp. 261–269; 279–281.
Goldman and Cohen, *Periodontal Therapy,* pp. 209–220.
Steele, *Dimensions of Dental Hygiene,* pp. 355–364.
Wilkins, *Clinical Practice of the Dental Hygienist,* pp. 151–154; 156–161.

READING ASSIGNMENTS FOR ENRICHMENT *

Steele, *Dimensions of Dental Hygiene*

pp. 166–167, 171–172 (Detecting Calculus with the Mirror and Explorer)
pp. 169–171 (Detecting Periodontal Pockets with the Periodontal Probe)
pp. 168–169 (Using Compressed Air)

Wilkins, *Clinical Practice of the Dental Hygienist*

pp. 198–199, 200–201 (Detecting Calculus with the Mirror and Explorer)
pp. 108–109, 138–139, 199–200 (Detecting Periodontal Pockets with the Periodontal Probe)
 p. 109 (Using Compressed Air)
pp. 201–202 (Detecting Calculus on Radiographs)

* See bibliography on page 252 for complete identification of publications listed here.

MODULE III

The Removal of Light to Moderate Calculus

1. PREREQUISITES

Before beginning work on this module, you must have successfully completed Modules I and II. Completing the exercises and review questions in this module requires the background knowledge provided by the earlier lessons. If you have not completed the previous modules, you will find it difficult to understand the instructions and perform the skills throughout this module.

2. PERFORMANCE OBJECTIVES

A. GENERAL OBJECTIVE

Given a mirror, explorer, curette, straight sickle, modified sickle, a fellow-student patient, and a manikin, the student will be able to demonstrate the technique for removal of light to moderate calculus.

161

B. SPECIFIC OBJECTIVES

Without the aid of source materials, the student must be able to:

1) demonstrate the use of the mirror and curette in the mouth of a fellow-student patient or on a manikin; appropriate mirror and instrument fulcrums, insertion, angulation, and strokes must be demonstrated on:

(a) all of the surfaces accessible from the buccal aspect of any posterior area designated by the instructor (posterior-most molar to first bicuspid).

(b) all of the surfaces accessible from the lingual aspect in this same area.

(c) all of the distal surfaces of the teeth in this same area using the opposite cutting edge of the blade.

(d) the labial aspect of either the maxillary or the mandibular anterior teeth using the correct working ends for the surfaces away from you and toward you.

2) demonstrate the use of the mirror and straight sickle on the lingual surfaces of the mandibular anterior teeth of a fellow-student patient or a manikin.

3) demonstrate the use of the modified sickle on the interproximal surfaces of any posterior area on a manikin.

3. DIRECTIONS FOR USE OF THE MODULE

The following are required for the successful completion of this module:

a dental mirror
a curette
a straight sickle
a modified sickle
a fellow-student patient or manikin

If you are going to work on a fellow-student patient, make sure that all of your instruments have been sterilized. When you are ready to perform the step-by-step procedures, have your patient hold up the copy of the module so that you can read the steps and refer to the photographs as you work in her mouth. If you are working on a manikin, set it up at your lab station and place the instruments on the desk next to the module.

Unlike in the previous modules, the review questions in this module are to be answered immediately after the performance checks. When you have successfully completed a performance check, answer the review questions and verify them with the Answer Key. When you are able to answer all of the questions correctly, go on to the next Skills Lesson.

4. SKILLS LESSONS

Lesson A: *Removing Calculus with the Curette*

Before discussing the use of the curette, it is important that we review the objective of scaling and the design of the curette. In order to restore the periodontal tissues to health, all soft and hard deposits must be removed from all surfaces coronal to the epithelial attachment on every tooth. To accomplish this goal, you have learned in the previous modules that *the most effective of all scaling instruments is the curette.*

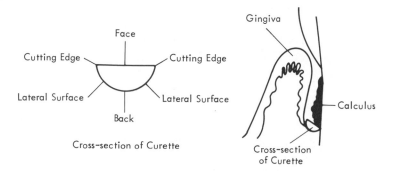

The curette is an instrument whose cutting edge is formed by the junction of the face and the curved lateral surface of the blade. The lateral surfaces extend from each cutting edge and curve around to merge and form the convex back of the blade. This is significant because when the cutting edge of the instrument is adapted to the tooth surface at the working angulation (45 to 90 degrees), *the rounded back of the blade is in contact with the sulcular epithelium.* The curette is the only scaling instrument that possesses this important feature of design. This allows the instrument to be inserted to the epithelial attachment without causing trauma. This capability is especially important for both deep and definitive scaling.

The curette is usually smaller and thinner than other scaling instruments and therefore permits better tactile sensitivity. Its small size and rounded back also allow it to be inserted easily under firm tissue or into deep narrow pockets. The curved cutting edges of the curette are more easily adapted to the curved tooth surfaces than the straight cutting edges of the sickles, hoes, and files. Also, the rounded toe of the curette is an important safety feature that the other instruments lack. The sickles, hoes, and files all have the disadvantage of possessing sharp corners and points on their blades that can gouge the cemental surface or the sulcular epithelium.

Curettes may vary in blade size, shank angulation and length, and handle size. All of these will be discussed in detail in MODULE V: Root Planing Procedure.

You have already had some experience in activating strokes with the curette in MODULE I. Then, in MODULE II you learned the finger rests for the different areas of the mouth. Now you will combine these skills and learn to use the curette in all areas of the mouth. In previous exercises use of the curette was limited to the buccal and mesial surfaces of the mandibular right posterior teeth. Now you must learn to use the curette on the distal surfaces as well.

There are three ways in which the curette may be used to scale the distal surfaces of the posterior teeth:

1) *You may use the working end that adapts to the distal surfaces of a quadrant.* If you are using an intraoral finger rest, this technique is really effective only on the bicuspids. If you attempt to use this technique on the molars with an intraoral finger rest, you will find it difficult to achieve working angulation because positioning the handle of the instrument parallel with the long axis of the tooth is close to impossible. When using this technique, it may be necessary to employ an extraoral finger rest to achieve proper angulation. The photographs below show that proper angulation can be achieved with this working end only when the handle is parallel to the long axis of the tooth. Can you see how the opposite arch would interfere with this ideal handle position on the molars and prohibit good working angulation?

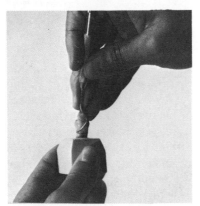 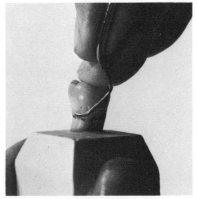

2) *You may use the working end that adapts to the mesial surfaces of a quadrant if you use the opposite cutting edge of the blade,* i.e., the cutting edge which is next to the tissue when the blade is adapted to the mesial surface.

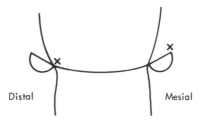

Distal   Mesial

The illustration above shows cross sections of the same blade as it is adapted to the mesial and distal surfaces of a molar. The X's show that the cutting edge, which is next to the tissue on the mesial (opposite cutting edge), can also be adapted to the distal. The photographs below show this technique. Notice that the *handle must be lowered* in order to achieve proper working angulation when the opposite cutting edge is adapted to the distal surface of the tooth. This position of the handle allows the use of an intraoral finger rest and makes this technique more practical and more effective than the one previously described.

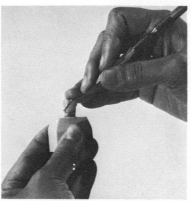
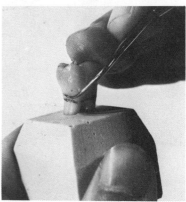

3) *You may use a curette that is designed to be adapted to distal surfaces only.* An instrument with a long contra-angled shank would permit easy access to the distal surfaces. The Gracey 13-14 curette is a commonly used instrument of this type.

Adaptation and Angulation for Distals

The following exercise will teach you to use the opposite cutting edge to scale the distal surface of the mandibular right first molar. You may practice on a fellow-student patient or a manikin. If you are working on a patient, position her, wash your hands, and begin working with sterile instruments. However, for the sake of clarity, the photographs for this exercise show the curette being used on a manikin.

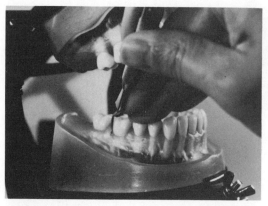

1. Establish your finger rest on the occlusal surfaces of the mandibular right bicuspids. Insert the curette at the distal line angle with a short, oblique stroke. Then position the handle so that it is as close to parallel with the long axis of the tooth as possible.

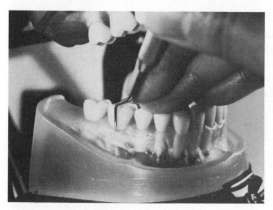

2. Activate exploratory strokes across the buccal surface by rotating your wrist slightly from left to right or by lowering your wrist and rocking back on your finger rest.

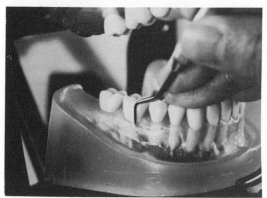

3. As you approach the mesial line angle, roll the handle from left to right in your fingers to keep the cutting edge adapted to the tooth surface.

If you do not keep the cutting edge well adapted, the toe of the curette will jut out into the tissue and lacerate it.

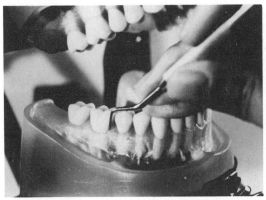

4. Lower your wrist and rock back on your finger rest to activate strokes across the mesial surface. Be sure to extend your strokes at least halfway across the mesial surface.

Withdraw the curette blade from the sulcus, but do not move on to the next tooth.

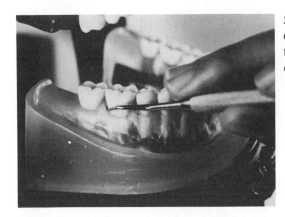

5. Maintain your finger rest on the bicuspids and roll the handle slightly counterclockwise until the opposite cutting edge of the blade is next to the tooth.

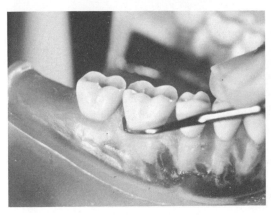

6. Adapt the opposite cutting edge just above the free margin in the area of the distal line angle. You should be able to see the face of the blade. Try raising and lowering the handle. *Can you see the angulation close as you lower the handle?*

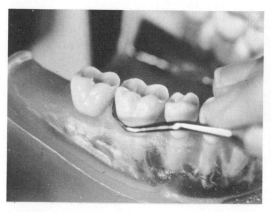

7. Lower the handle and close angulation to 0 degrees. Now insert the blade by slipping it under the free margin at the distal line angle. Insert it with an oblique stroke, pivoting on your finger rest from right to left.

Establish working angulation by raising your wrist slightly after you have reached the epithelial attachment.

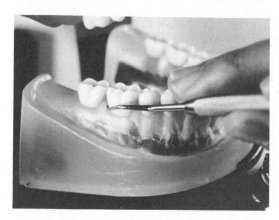

8. Lower your wrist and rock back on your finger rest to activate short, exploratory strokes across the distal surface. As you complete each stroke, your curette handle should be nearly *perpendicular* to the long axis of the tooth.

Now try moving on to the bicuspids. This technique works well on the bicuspids, but remember that you may use the other working end (that end that adapts to the distal surfaces in this quadrant) to scale the distal surfaces of these teeth because access is not so difficult. Try scaling the distal surfaces of the bicuspids with both techniques. Remember that one technique requires that the handle be nearly parallel with the tooth and the other requires that it be nearly perpendicular.

When you have practiced using the curette on the buccal aspect of the mandibular right posterior area, move on to the lingual surfaces of these same teeth. Scale the distal surfaces with the opposite cutting edge from the lingual aspect also. When you are confident of your skill, request a performance check.

Adaptation and Angulaton on Anteriors

The next exercise provides instructions for using the curette on the maxillary and mandibular anterior teeth. The object of the exercise is to teach you to use the correct working ends on the surfaces away from you and the surfaces toward you.

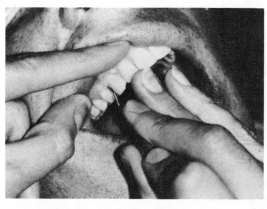

1. Retract the upper lip with your left index finger and establish your finger rest on the labio-incisal surfaces of the lateral and central incisors.

Begin scaling the surfaces toward you, starting with the distal surface of the right cuspid. Scaling of the labial surfaces may be accomplished by beginning strokes for the surfaces toward you just to the right of the midline of the labial surface. Then, when you are scaling the surfaces away from you, start your strokes just to the left of the midline to insure efficiency.

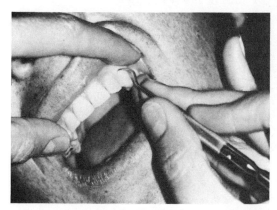

2. Scale all of the surfaces toward you, up to and including the mesial surface of the left cuspid. Keep moving your finger rest so that it is always to the right of your instrument.

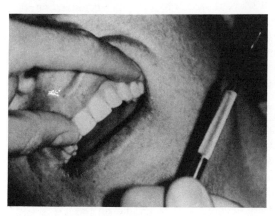

3. When you have finished scaling the mesial surface of the left cuspid, you must turn the instrument over if it is double-ended, or select its paired instrument if it is single-ended. *You must change working ends at this point in order to begin scaling the surfaces away from you.*

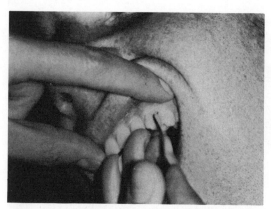

4. Insert your curette just to the left of the midline of the left cuspid and scale the labial and distal surfaces.

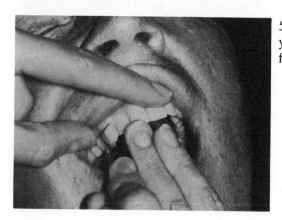

5. Scale all of the surfaces away from you, up to and including the mesial surface of the right cuspid.

Now repeat this exercise on the labial surfaces of the mandibular anterior teeth. When you are confident of your skill, request a performance check.

Now that you have learned to use the curette on the distal surfaces of posterior teeth and on the anteriors, you are almost ready to begin practicing the use of this instrument in all of the different areas of the mouth, as you did with the explorer. Before proceeding, let's review the following important keys to the effective use of the curette:

1) Remember to keep the handle as close to parallel with the tooth as possible. This will facilitate proper angulation of the blade and insure safe positioning of the toe of the instrument in the area of the epithelial attachment. The blade of a well designed curette should be directly in line with the long axis of its handle; therefore, as the handle is moved, the position of the blade and its cutting edges should be noted. The drawings below show the advantage of this technique. The handle on the left is well positioned for vertical or oblique strokes. The position of the handle on the right will permit only horizontal strokes with the sharp toe of the instrument pointed down toward the unprotected epithelial attachment.

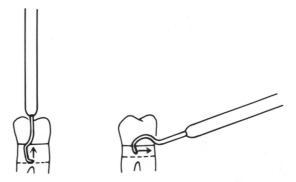

2) Constantly be aware of the angulation of your blade. With angulation for insertion, angulation for working strokes, and the undulant contours of the teeth to contend with, angulation is ever changing. Errors in angulation can result in trauma to the tissues as well as incomplete calculus removal. Remember to close your blade angulation to 0 degrees for insertion, or you may cause discomfort or lacerate the tissue as shown in the drawings below.

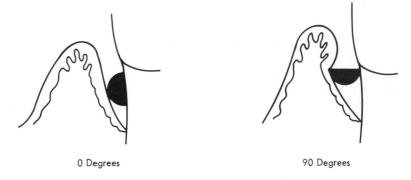

0 Degrees   90 Degrees

3) Roll the handle of your instrument in your fingers as you go over convexities and concavities in order to keep the cutting edge adapted to the tooth. Always visualize what the toe of your curette and the last few millimeters of cutting edge next to the toe are doing. The length of the cutting edge, including those few millimeters, must be in contact with the tooth and not jutting out into the tissue. Be careful not to roll the handle too much, or you will end up with only the toe in contact with the tooth. Can you see this in the illustrations below?

Not Rolled Enough   Correct   Rolled Too Much

4) When working on the lingual surfaces, keep the handle of your curette lingual to the tooth you are scaling to insure maintenance of proper angulation. If you are scaling a lingual surface and your curette handle is buccal to the tooth, only the toe of your curette, rather than the cutting edge, will be in contact with the lingual suface. This will result in ineffective calculus removal, scratching or gouging of the tooth surface, and distension and possible laceration of the tissue.

5) You have learned the positions of the basic fulcrums up to this point. Because you are now dealing with a curette, which involves not only adaptation but also angulation of a cutting edge, it will be necessary to modify your fulcrums slightly. Keep in mind that your wrist and finger motions must work in unison. This is where the correct choice of finger rest areas becomes critical. An excellent example of modifying a finger rest is the procedure one employs when working on the linguals of the lower right side. As you begin distal to the disto-lingual line angle, your fulcrum may be on the lower left. (As mentioned above, when working on the lingual surfaces, the handle of your instrument must be lingual to the tooth being scaled.) As you continue strokes onto the lingual surface, your fulcrum may move closer to the midline. Once you have begun scaling the mesial surface, your fulcrum moves to the lower right bicuspids. Another example of when fulcrum adaptation may be utilized is on the labial aspect of the upper anteriors. In the early part of the module, it was suggested that the fulcrum always be to the right of the working area. You may decide to place your fulcrum on the right or on the left, depending on the depth, and patient and operator positioning.

Performance Checklist for Lesson A: Removing Calculus with the Curette

Name _____

School _____

Date _____

	#1		#2	
	SATISFACTORY	UNSATISFACTORY	SATISFACTORY	UNSATISFACTORY
1. Demonstrate the appropriate mirror and instrument fulcrums, insertion, angulation and strokes with the curette on: a. all of the surfaces accessible from the buccal aspect of any posterior area designated by the instructor.				
b. all of the surfaces accessible from the lingual aspect in this same area.				
c. all of the distal surfaces of the teeth in this same area using the opposite cutting edge of the blade.				

Instructor _____

Performance Check Time _____

Comments: _____

_____

_____

_____

Now that you know the "do's" and "don'ts" for the use of the curette, practice using it in all areas of the mouth, beginning with the buccal aspect of the mandibular right posterior teeth. Follow the same sequence that you did when you worked with the explorer. You should be familiar with most of the finger rests by now, but it is advisable to refer back to MODULE II for specific positions and finger rests. The Performance Checklists for this lesson have covered only the use of the curette on the distal surfaces of the posteriors and on the anteriors; however, you should take full advantage of all the practice time allotted for use of the curette, because this will be the most important and most consistently used instrument in your armamentarium when you begin treating patients in the clinic. Your proficiency with this instrument is critical to your success as a dental hygienist. Use the knowledge and skill you have acquired from these modules as a springboard for perfecting your technique with the curette during the remainder of your dental hygiene education.

Review Questions for Lesson A: Removing Calculus with the Curette

Circle the letter of the *one* phrase which best completes the sentence.

1. The best instrument for removal of calculus located at the epithelial attachment is the:
    a. hoe
    b. sickle
    c. curette
    d. file
    e. chisel

2. The correct angulation of the curette for the removal of calculus is:
    a. more than 40 degrees, but less than 15 degrees
    b. less than 90 degrees, but more than 45 degrees
    c. more than 90 degrees, but less than 45 degrees
    d. less than 100 degrees

3. The curette may be inserted to the epithelial attachment with minimal tissue trauma because its blade:
    a. has a rounded back
    b. is easy to sharpen
    c. has rounded cutting edges
    d. provides good tactile sensitivity

4. The opposite cutting edge of a curette blade that is adapted to the mesial surface is that edge that is:
    a. closest to the buccal surface
    b. resting on the epithelial attachment
    c. next to the tooth
    d. next to the tissue

5. Label the indicated areas in this illustration of the curette blade.

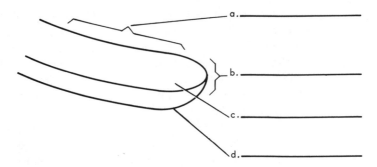

6. The curette permits better tactile sensitivity than other scaling instruments because its blade:

    a. is made of a different metal alloy
    b. has a longer cutting edge
    c. is usually smaller and thinner
    d. has a curved toe

The following illustrations show the curette blade in relation to a root during scaling. Examine them carefully before answering the next four questions.

7. Which drawing shows incorrect blade placement caused by failure to roll the instrument handle at the line angle?

  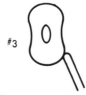

    a. Drawing #1
    b. Drawing #2
    c. Drawing #3
    d. Drawing #4

8. Incorrect blade placement of this type could result in:

    a. gouging of the tooth surface
    b. efficient removal of calculus
    c. tissue laceration with the toe
    d. effective soft tissue curettage
    e. all of the above

9. Which drawing shows incorrect blade placement caused by excessive rolling of the instrument handle at the line angle?

    a. Drawing #1
    b. Drawing #2
    c. Drawing #3
    d. Drawing #4

10. Incorrect blade placement of this type could result in:

    a. gouging of the root surface

    b. distension of the tissue

    c. laceration of the tissue

    d. discomfort to the patient

    e. all of the above

11. When scaling the distal surface of the mandibular right first molar with the opposite cutting edge of the blade, the handle of the instrument should be close to:

    a. parallel with the long axis of the tooth

    b. perpendicular to the long axis of the tooth

    c. 90 degrees to a horizontal plane

    d. parallel with the maxillary first molar

12. When working on a lingual surface, how should you position the curette handle to achieve the best angulation?

    a. perpendicular to the long axis of the tooth

    b. parallel with the long axis of the tooth

    c. buccal to the tooth

    d. lingual to the tooth

    e. a and c

    f. b and d

13. Which of these is not a method of scaling the distal surfaces of the posterior teeth?

    a. use the opposite cutting edge of the working end that adapts to the mesial surfaces of a quadrant

    b. use the opposite cutting edge of the working end that adapts to the distal surfaces of a quadrant

    c. use the working end that adapts to the distal surfaces of a quadrant

    d. use a curette that is designed to adapt to distal surfaces only

14. After scaling the surfaces of the anterior teeth toward you, what must you do in order to scale the surfaces away from you?

    a. switch to an extraoral fulcrum

    b. lower your instrument handle

    c. use the opposite cutting edge of the same blade

    d. change working ends

    e. recontour your blade by sharpening

15. Correct angulation of insertion of the curette is:

    a. 0 degrees

    b. 45 degrees

    c. 0–45 degrees

    d. 90 degrees

    e. 45–90 degrees

Correct your answers with the Answer Key on page 191.

Performance Checklist for Lesson A: Removing Calculus with the Curette

Name _____

School _____

Date _____

	#1		#2	
	SATISFACTORY	UNSATISFACTORY	SATISFACTORY	UNSATISFACTORY
2. Demonstrate the appropriate mirror and instrument fulcrums, insertion, angulation, and strokes with the curette on the labial or lingual aspect of either the maxillary or the mandibular anterior teeth, using the current working ends for the surfaces away from you and toward you.				

Instructor _____

Performance Check Time _____

Comments: _____

_____

_____

_____

Lesson B: Removing Calculus with the Straight Sickle

The *straight sickle* has two straight cutting edges, each of which is formed by the junction of its face and a flat side. The sides join to form the sharp, pointed back of the instrument. This gives the sickle its characteristic triangular cross section. However, some manufacturers produce sickles with flattened backs as illustrated below.

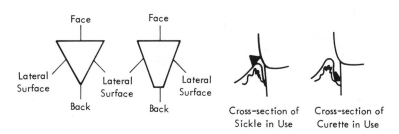

The design of the sickle differs from that of the curette, whose sides are curved and merge to form a convex back. When the curette is inserted subgingivally, its rounded back comes into contact with the sulcular epithelium, allowing the instrument to be lowered to the epithelial attachment without its causing trauma to the tissue. This is especially important for both deep and definitive scaling. On the other hand, the sickle cannot be inserted to the epithelial attachment without trauma because in the course of insertion its back will lacerate the sulcular tissue. For this reason, the sickle can only be used for removal of supragingival deposits or for removal of those deposits that extend slightly below the free margin of gingiva if the tissue is distensible enough to permit insertion.

The flat sides of the sickle are tapered to form a pointed end, which can easily cause trauma to the tissue if it is inserted subgingivally. This is due to the fact that (unlike the curette whose cutting edges are curved) the straight cutting edges of the sickle cannot be adapted to the curved contours of the tooth.

Sickles generally have larger, heavier blades than curettes. This decreases tactile sensitivity. The blade, shank, and handle of the straight sickle are all on the same plane and therefore are reserved for scaling anterior teeth. When the blade is applied to the tooth, the angle between the instrument's face and the tooth should be less than 90 degrees, but more than 45 degrees. The calculus deposit is engaged and removed with a pull stroke.

Since the straight sickle is used almost exclusively for the removal of supragingival calculus on the anterior teeth (especially on the linguals of the mandibular anteriors), the following exercise demonstrates the use of the instrument in this particular area. For the sake of photographic clarity, the instrument shown in the following pictures is being used on a manikin.

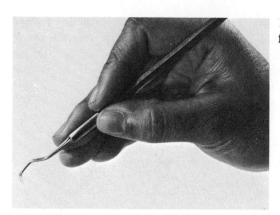

1. Hold the straight sickle with a modified pen grasp.

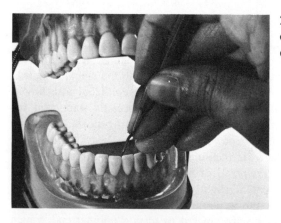

2. Establish your finger rest on the incisal surfaces of the mandibular left lateral and cuspids.

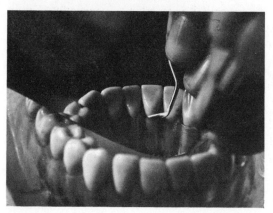

3. Begin scaling the lingual surface of the left central by placing the cutting edge just above the free margin. Make sure that the sharp pointed tip and the straight cutting edge are well adapted to the tooth. If you adapt the center of the cutting edge rather than the last few millimeters adjacent to the pointed tip, you will surely lacerate the marginal gingival.

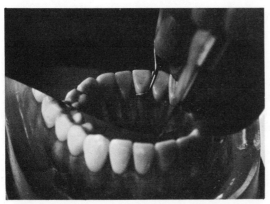

4. Scale the mesial surface. Be sure to use short strokes—extending from the free margin upward. Watch the back of the blade as well as the tip to make sure that you are not lacerating the marginal gingiva or the papilla.

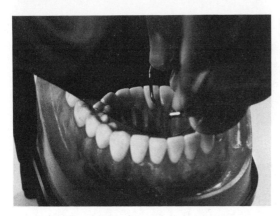

5. Now scale the distal surface. You may wish to do this from a back position because it is difficult to scale the surfaces away from you from a side position.

Practice using the straight sickle on the mandibular anteriors and then go on to the exercise for modified sickles. When you have practiced using both instruments and are ready for your performance check, notify your instructor.

Lesson C: *Removing Calculus with the Modified Sickle*

The *modified sickle* was designed so that the sickle scaler could be adapted to posterior teeth. To accomplish this, a contra-angle bend is added to the shank so that the blade, shank, and handle are not in the same plane as they are in the straight sickle. Otherwise, the modified sickle and the straight sickle are identical in design and have the same limitations. Straight and modified sickles should be classed with the hoes and files as gross scalers, and are not suitable for definitive scaling. If the modified sickle is utilized to remove subgingival calculus, it should be applied only to those deposits extending just below the free margin of gingiva where the tissue is distensible enough to permit its insertion. It should never be inserted to the epithelial attachment.

Use of the modified sickle is followed by use of curettes for final calculus removal and smoothing of the root surface.

In this exercise you will practice using the modified sickle for removing supragingival calculus and gross subgingival calculus. Begin working on the mandibular right second molar.

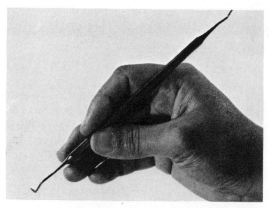

1. Hold the modified sickle with a modified pen grasp.

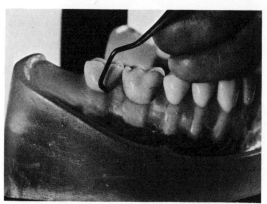

2. Adapt the appropriate blade to the mesial line angle of the mandibular right second molar. Place the cutting edge just above the free margin, taking care not to allow the back or pointed tip of the blade to harm the tissue.

If you are scaling supragingival calculus, begin activating short strokes in the area above the free margin by lowering your wrist and rocking back on your finger rest.

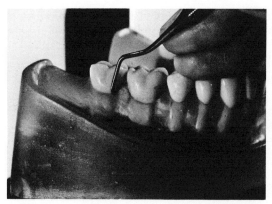

3. If you are planning to remove a sub-gingival ledge of calculus, carefully insert the blade at the mesial line angle. Watch the back of the blade very carefully as the blade is inserted. Do not attempt to insert this instrument to the epithelial attachment. Insert to get under a calculus ledge only when the tissue in the area is easily displaced.

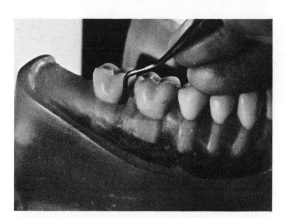

4. Scale the mesial surface by lowering your wrist and rocking back on your finger rest. Carefully withdraw the blade from the sulcus by first coming up to the contact area and then pulling out.

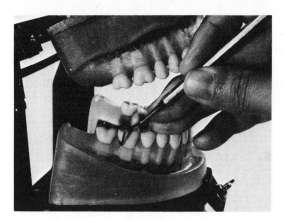

5. Now adapt the other working end of the modified sickle to the distal line angle of the first molar. Make sure that the cutting edge is well adapted from the tip of the instrument to about the center of the cutting edge.

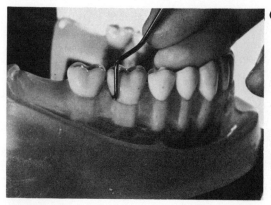

6. Insert the blade at the distal line angle.

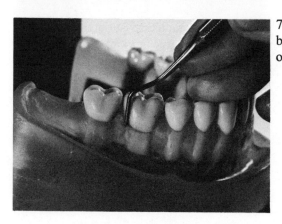

7. Activate strokes on the distal surface by lowering your wrist and rocking back on your finger rest.

When you have practiced using both the straight and the modified sickle to your satisfaction, ask your instructor for a performance check.

Review Questions for Lesson B: Removing Calculus with the Straight Sickle and Lesson C: Removing Calculus with the Modified Sickle

1. The straight sickle should *not* be used for:
   a. removal of supragingival calculus on the linguals of the mandibular anteriors
   b. removal of stain and calculus in the fossae of the maxillary anteriors
   c. removal of supragingival calculus from the interproximals of the mandibular anteriors
   d. removal of subgingival calculus on the mandibular anteriors

2. The cutting edges of sickle scalers are formed by the junction of:
   a. two flat surfaces (face and side)
   b. two curved surfaces (face and side)
   c. a curved side and a flat face
   d. a curved face and a flat side

3. The modified sickle is designed primarily for use on the:
    a. interproximals of anterior teeth
    b. lingual and buccal surfaces
    c. lingual calculus on the mandibular anteriors
    d. interproximals of the posterior teeth
    e. distals of molars

4. Which of the following is true of the sickle scaler?
    a. it is not suitable for heavy calculus
    b. it allows very good tactile sensitivity
    c. it is difficult to adapt to curved surfaces
    d. it is always used subgingivally on anteriors

5. Which design feature(s) of the sickle limit(s) its use in subgingival areas?
    a. sharp, pointed tip
    b. straight cutting edges
    c. sharp back of the blade
    d. bulky blade
    e. c and d
    f. all of the above

Performance Checklist for Lesson B: Removing Calculus with the Straight Sickle
and Lesson C: Removing Calculus with the Modified Sickle

Name _____

School _____

Date _____

	#1		#2	
	SATISFACTORY	UNSATISFACTORY	SATISFACTORY	UNSATISFACTORY
3. Demonstrate the use of the mirror and straight sickle on the lingual surfaces of the mandibular anterior teeth.				
4. Demonstrate the use of the modified sickle on the interproximal surfaces of any posterior area.				

Instructor _____

Performance Check Time _____

Comments: _____

_____

_____

ANSWER KEY

LESSON A

1. c
2. b
3. a
4. d
5. a—cutting edge
   b—face or facial surface
   c—toe
   d—back
6. c
7. b
8. c
9. c

10. e
11. b
12. f
13. b
14. d
15. a

LESSON B

1. d
2. a
3. d
4. c
5. f

READING ASSIGNMENTS FOR ENRICHMENT *

Goldman and Cohen, *Periodontal Therapy:*
     pp. 391–395 (Removing Calculus with the Curette)
     pp. 391; 409 (Removing Calculus with the Straight and Modified Sickles)

Steele, *Dimensions of Dental Hygiene:*
     pp. 180–183 (Removing Calculus with the Curette)
     pp. 186–188 (Removing Calculus with the Straight and Modified Sickles)

Wilkins, *Clinical Practice of the Dental Hygienist:*
     pp. 183–184, 207–208 (Removing Calculus with the Curette)
     pp. 180–182, 204–205 (Removing Calculus with the Straight and Modified Sickles)

     * See bibliography on page 252 for complete identification of publications listed here.

MODULE IV

The Removal of Heavy Calculus

1. PREREQUISITES

Before beginning work on this module, you must have successfully completed modules I through III, which comprise part one of the unit: The Detection and Removal of Calculus.

2. PERFORMANCE OBJECTIVES

A. GENERAL OBJECTIVE

Given a set of hoes, a set of files, one or two extracted teeth with calculus, and a manikin, the student will be able to demonstrate the use of these instruments for the removal of heavy calculus.

B. SPECIFIC OBJECTIVES

Without the aid of source materials, the student will be able to:

193

1) plan and record the sequence of procedures for a series of appointments for a hypothetical patient who has heavy calculus.

2) demonstrate the techniques for removal of gross calculus from the distal, lingual, and mesial surfaces of an extracted tooth using the hoes.

3) demonstrate the use of hoes on four surfaces (distal, buccal, mesial, and lingual) of the mandibular right first molar of the manikin.

4) demonstrate the technique for removal of gross calculus from distal, buccal, and mesial surfaces of an extracted tooth using files.

5) demonstrate the use of files on four surfaces (distal, buccal, mesial and lingual) of the mandibular right first molar of the manikin.

6) describe the advantages and disadvantages of the use of ultrasonic scaling devices.

7) describe the procedure for applying a topical anesthetic.

8) describe the indications and contraindications for the use of local anesthesia in scaling.

9) describe the postoperative instructions that apply specifically to a patient after scaling of heavy calculus.

3. DIRECTIONS FOR USE OF THE MODULE

The following materials and equipment are required for the successful completion of this module:

a set of hoes
a set of files
one or two extracted molars mounted in stone *
a dental manikin, preferably with randomly applied artificial calculus *

The manikin should be set up at the lab station and adjusted according to directions from your instructor. All other materials and equipment should be laid out on the desk next to the module.

At the end of each Skills Lesson in this module, you will answer review questions pertaining to the particular skill that had just been described. When you are able to answer all questions correctly and perform the skill, ask for an evaluation. If your instructor is occupied and cannot check you immediately, you may go on to the next Skills Lesson while you are waiting. As you demonstrate the skills listed on the Performance Checklist, the instructor will evaluate and record your performance. If your ratings are all satisfactory, proceed to the next Skills Lesson. If any

---

* These items will be issued by the instructor.

of your ratings are unsatisfactory, review the exercise(s) and request another performance check when you are ready.

It must be emphasized that despite all efforts, no textbook, illustration, audiovisual aid, or other instructional material can render sufficient instruction by itself in the field of dental hygiene. The degree of skill necessary to provide quality dental care cannot be attained without the guidance and critical observation of qualified, concerned instructors.

The modules in this unit provide individualized instruction and can be most effectively utilized when each one is used as a "cookbook." As gourmet chefs work in the kitchen, following recipes that include specific ingredients and instructions, the dental hygiene student should work with modules in the laboratory or clinic following detailed procedure "recipes" that include important concepts and key steps. Leaving out an ingredient in a recipe or measuring that ingredient inaccurately may result in a culinary disaster. In this unit, failure to complete any exercise, reading assignment, or test will result in less than quality care for your patients in the clinic.

Excellent comprehension of all concepts and skills in a module is imperative because each module builds upon the previous one. In order to derive the full benefit of this type of instruction, it is of utmost importance that the student carefully follow each set of instructions.

4. SKILLS LESSONS

***Lesson A:** Planning the Sequence of Procedures for a Series of Appointments*

Patients with any degree of periodontal disease, from acute gingivitis to severe periodontitis, often require a series of appointments. Multiple appointments are essential to accomplish thorough scaling and to determine tissue response. The number of appointments required is dependent on the amount, tenacity, and mode of attachment of the calculus; type of cementum (normal or necrotic); degree of pathology and depth of pockets; patient's home care; and operator's skill.

There may be many different indications for scheduling more than one appointment for your patient. He may have moderate to heavy calculus; painful, edematous, and hemorrhagic tissue due to heavy plaque or acute necrotizing ulcerative gingivitis (ANUG)); root surfaces that require extensive planing; or he may simply need a check-up on his home care and tissue response. The hygienist's ability to plan treatment requires judgment based on knowledge, experience, and recognition of subtle changes in the periodontium. Initially, your decisions should be the result of faculty consultation.

Each scaling session should be as advantageous for the patient as possible. The majority of calculus must be removed at the initial gross scaling because the roughened surface of residual calculus harbors plaque that will retard healing. It is suggested that quadrant or arch scaling be scheduled when such a series of appointments is indicated.

Only the operator can determine the number of appointments necessary for thorough subgingival scaling. Minimal depth, confined areas of pathology, and minimal cemental irregularity may indicate only one appointment for root planing; whereas, a severely involved periodontal patient may require several appointments. You must evaluate your own capabilities to determine how much work you can accomplish in a given length of time (usually 45 minutes to an hour in private practice). You may need to schedule only two appointments, or you may plan to see the patient as many as eight times or more. A sequence of appointments should establish a systematic approach to insure thoroughness and to increase efficiency. Suggested sequences of procedures are listed below for various multiple appointment cases.

Two appointments

Appointment #1: Full mouth gross scaling
Appointment #2: Full mouth definitive scaling and root planing

Three appointments

Appointment #1: Gross scaling of maxillary arch or maxillary and mandibular right quadrants
Appointment #2: Gross scaling of mandibular arch or maxillary and mandibular left quadrants
Appointment #3: Full mouth definitive scaling and root planing

Four appointments

Appointment #1: Gross scaling of maxillary arch or maxillary and mandibular right quadrants
Appointment #2: Gross scaling of mandibular arch or maxillary and mandibular left quadrants
Appointment #3: Begin full mouth definitive scaling and root planing
Appointment #4: Complete full mouth definitive scaling and root planing

Five appointments

Appointment #1: Gross scaling of maxillary right quadrant
Appointment #2: Gross scaling of mandibular right quadrant
Appointment #3: Gross scaling of maxillary left quadrant
Appointment #4: Gross scaling of mandibular left quadrant
Appointment #5: Full mouth definitive scaling and root planing

These suggested sequences are only a few of the many possible series of appointments you might plan (with the help of your clinical instructor) for your patient. Multiple appointments offer a number of advantages to you as well as to your patient. This plan is a great aid to patient education because with it you can show him a comparison of the tissue on the second visit so that he can clearly see the difference. This comparison also allows you to judge the final outcome of the scaling by the tissue response. Furthermore, for the patient, it interrupts the stress of instrumentation and confines the sensitivity that may result on one side of the mouth. No matter how you sequence your procedures, always remember that all ledges and large pieces of calculus should be removed during gross scaling. Look at the patient's radiographs and examine his mouth carefully with the mirror and explorer for subgingival calculus—then decide how much you will attempt to accomplish during the first appointment. Do not attempt gross scaling of the entire mouth unless you are sure you will be able to do it thoroughly. It is far better to scale only one quadrant well than to attempt gross scaling of the entire mouth and fail to do a thorough job.

As a general rule, the final appointment with the patient should require only very fine scaling and root planing. If you are still doing heavy scaling at this point, reevaluate the case and extend the number of scaling appointments.

When scheduling a series of appointments, allow one week to elapse before re-scaling the same area to permit time for healing. This is particularly important when you have done gross scaling on the entire mouth during the initial appointment.

Patients should not be scheduled on a recall basis until all definitive scaling and root planing is completed, and home care is adequate. The first recall appointment should be scheduled within three months of the end of the first series of appointments so that you can evaluate the patient's periodontal condition and the effectiveness of his home care.

Review Questions for Lesson A: Planning a Sequence of Procedures

for a Series of Appointments

Circle the letter of the *one* best answer.

1. Nearly all calculus should be removed during gross scaling because roughened calculus:

    a. is harder to remove from root surfaces

    b. harbors plaque, which retards healing

    c. will scratch the sulcular epithelium

    d. will become embedded in cementum

2. Which of the following conditions might indicate that a patient requires more than one appointment?

    a. moderate supragingival and subgingival calculus

    b. moderate supragingival and heavy subgingival calculus

    c. inflamed, hemorrhagic tissue
    d. rough, exposed root surfaces
    e. all of the above
    f. a and b only

3. Set up a series of appointments for a patient who has heavy subgingival calculus in all posterior areas, moderate supragingival and subgingival calculus on the mandibular anteriors, and edematous, hemorrhagic tissue.

Appointment No.	*Date*	*Procedure*
#1	10–14–71	

4. The final appointment with a patient after a series of appointments should require only:
    a. final gross scaling
    b. subgingival scaling
    c. supragingival scaling
    d. fine scaling and root planing

5. The first recall appointment should be scheduled within:
    a. one month
    b. three months
    c. four months
    d. six months

See Answer Key on page 227 for correct responses.

Lesson B: Removing Calculus with the Hoe

The *hoe* is a scaler reserved for dislodging heavy supragingival and subgingival calculus in easily accessible areas. It is a bulky instrument whose single straight cutting edge is formed by the junction of the face and the bevelled toe of the blade. The blade of the hoe is angled at 99 to 100 degrees to the shank; the toe has a 45-degree bevel. The drawing on the right shows the hoe in cross section as it is placed subgingivally. You can see how the back of the blade would displace and injure the tissue if the cutting edge were placed at the epithelial attachment.

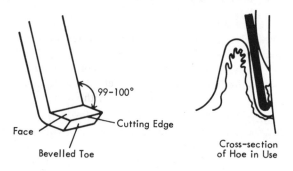

99–100°
Face
Cutting Edge
Bevelled Toe

Cross-section
of Hoe in Use

Hoes may be single- or double-ended. They are paired instruments, and a set of four working ends is required for the four surfaces of a tooth. In other words, there is a specific working end designed for each of four tooth surfaces: distal, buccal, mesial, and lingual. Hoes vary in shank angulation, shank length, and blade size. Hoes with long, angled shanks are designed for removing calculus ledges in the posterior areas. Because of blade size, adaptation to proximal surfaces is poor if not impossible. *Hoes are most effective when employed for buccal and lingual surfaces, or on proximal surfaces adjacent to edentulous areas.* Hoes whose shanks have little angulation are designed for anterior areas, again primarily for the labial and lingual surfaces. Because of the thickness of their blades, hoes lack adaptability and tactile sensitivity, and should be used subgingivally only when the tissue is easily displaced. *A good rule of thumb for the use of any instrument is not to force it subgingivally if it does not insert with ease.*

In addition to its inability to remove deposits at the epithelial attachment, the hoe is seriously limited in the poor adaptability of its straight cutting edge. When the straight cutting edge of the hoe is placed on a curved tooth surface such as a line angle, one sharp corner of the blade will gouge the root surface while the other gouges the sulcular epithelium. For this reason, only vertical strokes should be used. Oblique and horizontal strokes will increase the chances of trauma.

The hoe is only used with a pull stroke. The cutting edge should be angulated at 90 degrees to the tooth surface. Be sure proper angulation is established prior to activating your pull stroke. Improper angulation will cause the instrument to slip over and smooth or burnish the calculus.

When activating strokes, the instrument may contact the tooth surface at the cutting edge and again on the shank. This double contact serves to provide leverage and control for breaking off heavy deposits. As with instrumentation of all scalers used for gross calculus removal, instrumentation with the hoe must be followed by definitive scaling with the curette.

USE OF THE HOE ON AN EXTRACTED MOLAR

Before learning to use the hoe on the manikin, try removing some heavy calculus from the extracted molar and observe the effect of the straight cutting edge on the root surfaces. Because you may have only one molar with heavy calculus instead of two, the following exercise requires you to scale only one-half of the tooth. You will scale only the lingual surface, half of the mesial surface, and half of the distal surface with your hoes. The other half of the tooth should be reserved for the next lesson, which teaches the use of the file.

Note: With the hoes and files used in these photographs, proper adaptation demands that the shank immediately above the blade be parallel to the long axis of the tooth.

Buccal and Lingual

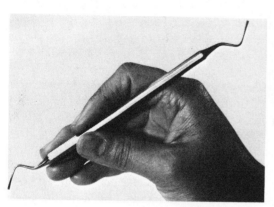

1. Select a hoe that is designed for the lingual surface of the mandibular left first molar. Hold the instrument with a modified pen grasp. The picture shows a double-ended hoe that has a working end for the buccal surfaces and one for the lingual surfaces on the same handle.

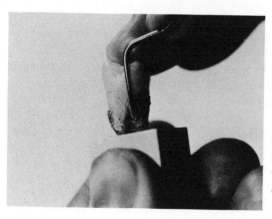

2. Hold the extracted molar with the lingual surface toward you and remove ledges and large pieces of calculus from the lingual surface. *Activate vertical strokes* by turning your wrist from left to right. Work until almost all of the calculus has been removed.

Examine the root surface while you are using the hoe and after you have finished with it. Observe the effects of the straight cutting edge on the cementum.

INTERPROXIMAL

3. Select the hoe designed for the mesial surfaces. Hold it with a modified pen grasp. This picture shows a double-ended hoe with working ends for the mesial and distal surfaces.

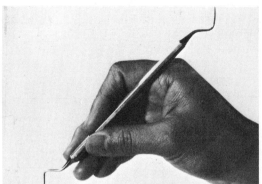

4. Remove all gross calculus from one half of either proximal surface. Extend your strokes only halfway across the surface.

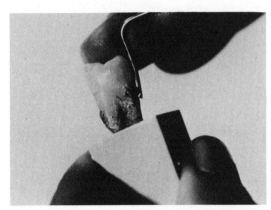

5. Use the hoe designed for the distal surfaces to remove half of the gross calculus on the other proximal surface. Again, extend your strokes only halfway across.

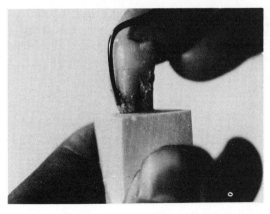

If you have two extracted molars with calculus, reserve one for the next lesson; then go ahead and remove all of the gross calculus from this molar with your hoes. Later, when you have done gross scaling on the other molar with the files, you can make a comparison between its cemental surfaces and those worked on with the hoes.

USE OF THE HOE ON A MANIKIN

Now, prepare to use the hoes on the mandibular right first and second molars of the manikin. You will be working on all four tooth surfaces, and so you will need a complete set of hoes for this exercise.

Buccal and Lingual

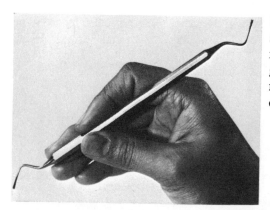

1. Select the hoe designed for the buccal surface of the mandibular right first molar. Hold the hoe with a modified pen grasp. (Notice that this same working end may also be adapted to the lingual surface of the mandibular left first molar.)

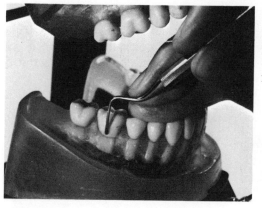

2. Establish your finger rest on the occlusal surfaces of the mandibular right bicuspids and gently place the blade against the buccal surface just above the free margin of the gingiva.

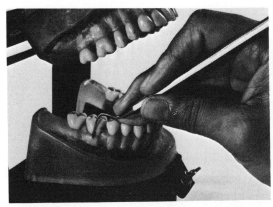

3. Carefully insert the hoe by first placing the bevelled toe of the blade flush against the tooth, just above the free margin, and then rotating your wrist from left to right while gently pushing the instrument apically.

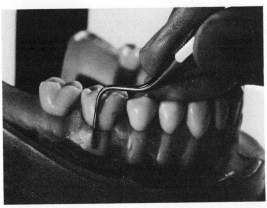

4. Insert the blade until the cutting edge is just below the ledge of calculus you wish to remove.

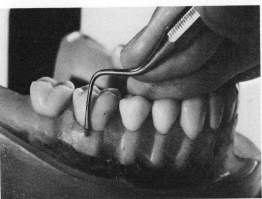

5. Establish blade angulation of about 90 degrees and activate vertical strokes to break the calculus ledge by lowering your wrist and rocking back on your finger rest. Continue using short, vertical strokes across the buccal surface.

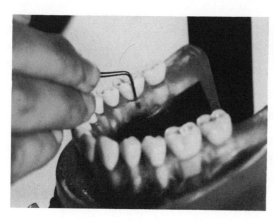

6. Select the hoe designed for the lingual surface of the mandibular right first molar and proceed to scale that surface.

INTERPROXIMAL

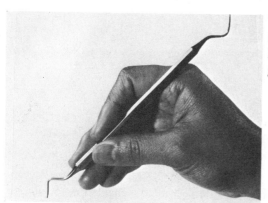

7. Select the hoe designed for the mesial surface of the mandibular right first molar. Hold the instrument with a modified pen grasp.

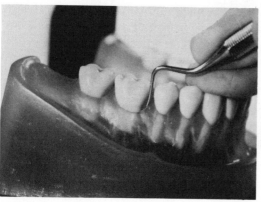

8. Carefully insert the hoe and scale the mesial surface of the molar by lowering your wrist and rocking back on your finger rest. Can you see how difficult it is to maintain good adaptation and angulation in this interproximal area? Because of this problem the hoe is rarely used on a proximal surface unless the adjacent space is edentulous.

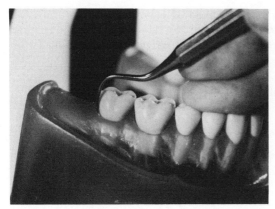

9. Insert the hoe on the distal surface of the posterior-most molar in the mandibular right quadrant. The hoe is very effective for breaking off heavy ledges of calculus in this area. Since there is no adjacent tooth, it is much easier to adapt the blade and activate vertical strokes.

Review Questions for Lesson B: Removing Calculus with the Hoe

1. A serious limitation of the hoes is that they:
   a. cannot remove calculus at the epithelial attachment
   b. are not designed for heavy calculus removal
   c. only adapt to buccal and mesial surfaces
   d. cannot be sharpened frequently

2. How many working ends of a hoe are needed to make a complete set that will adapt to all tooth surfaces?
   a. one working end
   b. two working ends
   c. three working ends
   d. four working ends
   e. six working ends

3. The hoe is used primarily for:
   a. detection of large calculus ledges
   b. removal of large supragingival deposits
   c. removal of limited amounts of subgingival calculus
   d. removal of calculus at the epithelial attachment
   e. a and c
   f. b and c

4. Which of the following is *not* true of the hoes?
   a. they have one straight cutting edge
   b. they have a series of cutting edges
   c. the blade is angulated 99 to 100 degrees to the shank
   d. they have sharp points that can traumatize tissue

5. Because hoes are not designed to adapt well to the tooth surface, their use is restricted to:
   a. buccal and lingual surfaces and proximal surfaces adjacent to edentulous areas

b. any proximal surface adjacent to an edentulous area
c. all surfaces of all the teeth
d. interproximal surfaces and the lingual surfaces of the mandibular anteriors.

See Answer Key on page 227 for correct responses.

Performance Checklist for Lesson B: Removing Calculus with the Hoe

Name _____

School _____

Date _____

	#1		#2	
	SATISFACTORY	UNSATISFACTORY	SATISFACTORY	UNSATISFACTORY
1. Demonstrate the technique for removal of gross calculus from the distal, lingual and mesial surfaces of an extracted tooth using hoes.				
2. Demonstrate the use of hoes on the four surfaces (distal, buccal, mesial and lingual) of the mandibular right first molar of the manikin.				

Instructor _____

Performance Check Time _____

Comments: _____

_____

_____

_____

Lesson C: *Removing Calculus with the File*

The *file* is a heavy instrument with multiple cutting edges. It is used to crush or fracture very heavy, tenacious calculus. Its blade size, lack of adaptability, and limited tactile sensitivity restrict its use to supragingival or subgingival areas where the tissue can easily be displaced.

The file consists of a series of blades on a base. Each blade in the series is identical to the blade of the hoe. Angulation of the blades in relation to the shank may be from 90 to 105 degrees. The base of the blades may be round, oval, or rectangular, and is an extension of the shank. Files may also vary in shank angulation and length. Shank variations are most critical where there is pocket depth and/or gingival recession. Generally, instruments used on posterior teeth have greater shank angulation than those used on the anteriors.

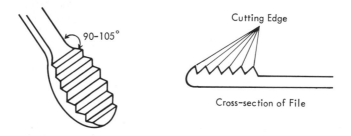

The file is most commonly used to crush heavy ledges of calculus on the dstal surface of the last molar. The file does *not* remove calculus completely when used in this manner. It merely *fractures* and *roughens* the surface of the calculus to allow easier removal with the curette. Like the hoes, these instruments are too large to be readily adapted to the interproximal areas. Instead they are best applied to buccal and lingual surfaces, and to surfaces adjacent to edentulous areas. Also, like the hoes, they are designed in sets of four working ends, one for each tooth surface.

Stabilization of this instrument for control must be emphasized. This may be accomplished by engaging the deposit with the cutting edges and resting the shank on the tooth. *Pull strokes* should be used to activate this instrument.

Since it is closely akin to the hoe in design, the file shares the limitations of the hoe. Care should be taken not to use excessive instrumentation with the file because adaptation of the straight cutting edges to curved surfaces is very poor. Severe gouging of the root surface and adjacent tissue may result unless all of the cutting edges are well adapted. The illustration below shows the file in cross section in a periodontal pocket. Like the hoe, this instrument cannot remove calculus at the epithelial attachment and therefore its use must be followed by that of the curette.

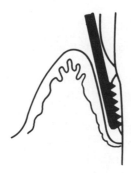

USE OF THE FILE ON AN EXTRACTED MOLAR

We will now use the files to repeat the same exercises you performed with the hoes. Work on the other half of the same extracted molar or use a new extracted molar if you have one.

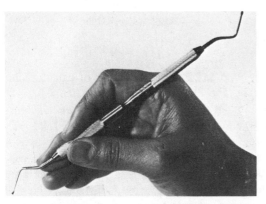

BUCCAL AND LINGUAL

1. Select the file that is designed for the buccal surface of the mandibular right first molar. Hold the instrument with a modified pen grasp. A double-ended file is shown here. It has one working end for the buccal surfaces and one for the lingual surfaces on the same handle.

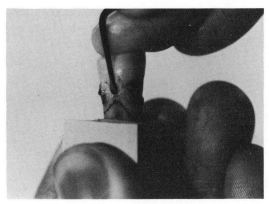

2. Hold the extracted molar with the buccal surface toward you and remove ledges and large pieces of calculus from the buccal surface. Activate vertical strokes by turning your wrist from left to right. When almost all of the calculus has been removed, examine the root surfaces to observe the effects of the multiple straight cutting edges of the file.

INTERPROXIMAL

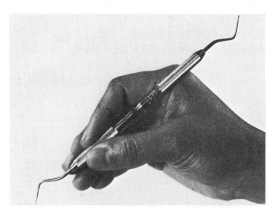

3. Select the file designed for the mesial surfaces. This picture shows a double-ended file for mesial and distal surfaces being held with a modified pen grasp.

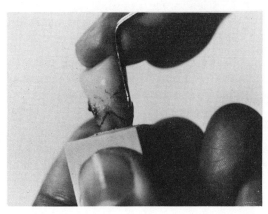

4. Remove all gross calculus from one-half of the mesial surface. Extend your strokes halfway across the surface. If you are using the same tooth you used with the hoes, the mesial surface should be completely free of gross calculus when you finish.

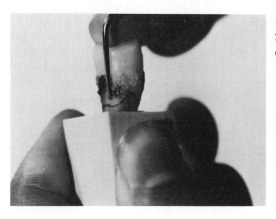

5. Use the file designed for the distal surfaces to remove the other half of the calculus left on the distal surface.

If you have an entire extracted molar to work on rather than just a half, continue to work on it with the files. When you have finished, compare those surfaces scaled with the files to those previously scaled with the hoes. Save these teeth for the next module on root planing. You will be using these teeth with their roughened root surfaces for the root planing exercises.

Now, let's move on to using the files on the manikin. As with the hoes, you will be working on four tooth surfaces.

USE OF THE FILE ON A MANIKIN

BUCCAL AND LINGUAL

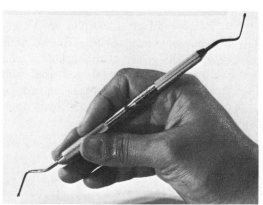

1. Select a file designed for the buccal surface of the mandibular right first molar. Hold it with a modified pen grasp.

Notice that this same working end may also be adapted to the lingual surface of the mandibular left first molar.

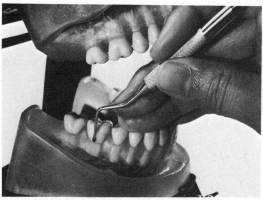

2. Establish your finger rest on the occlusal surfaces of the mandibular right bicuspids and place the blade gently against the buccal surface just above the free margin of the gingiva.

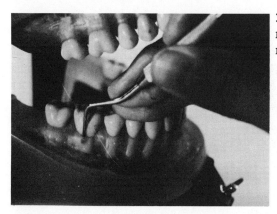

3. Carefully insert the file under the free margin by lifting your wrist slightly and rocking forward on your finger rest.

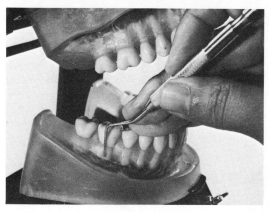

4. Gently push the file apically until the cutting edges engage the piece of calculus you wish to remove.

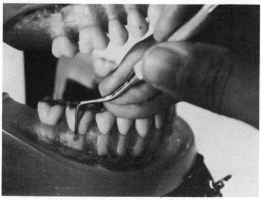

5. Adapt the head of the file against the deposit so the cutting edges "bite" into the calculus. Activate vertical strokes by lowering your wrist and rocking back on your finger rest. Continue using vertical strokes until the calculus has been crushed and its surface is rough. Remember that the file is used to break up large pieces or ledges of calculus to allow easy removal with the curette.

INTERPROXIMAL

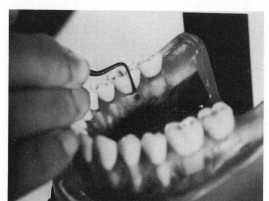

6. Select the file designed for the lingual surface of the mandibular right first molar and scale that surface as you did the buccal surface.

7. Select the file designed for the mesial surface of the mandibular right first molar and hold it with a modified pen grasp.

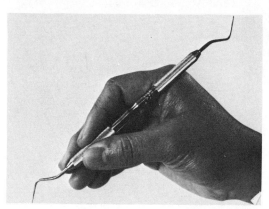

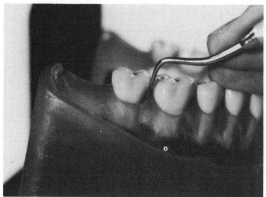

8. Carefully insert the file and scale the mesial surface by lowering your wrist and rocking back on your finger rest. As with the hoe, it is very difficult to achieve proper adaptation and angulation with the file in an interproximal area. This instrument is only used on proximal surfaces when the adjacent space is edentulous.

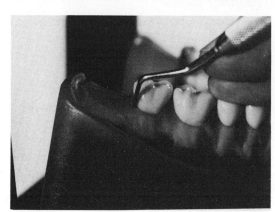

9. Insert the file on the distal surface of the posterior-most molar in the mandibular right quadrant. The file is often used to crush ledges of calculus in this area. Activate strokes here by lowering your wrist and rocking back on your finger rest.

Note: Hoes and files may be used on anterior teeth. The instrument used interproximally in the posterior area is used on the labial and lingual surfaces of the anteriors, while the instrument used bucco-lingually is adapted interproximally on the anteriors.

Review Questions for Lesson C: Removing Calculus with the File

1. Which of the following factors restricts the use of the file to supragingival areas or subgingival areas where the tissue is easily displaced?
    a. size of the blade
    b. straight cutting edges
    c. limited tactile sensitivity
    d. sharp corners on blade
    e. all of the above
2. The file is easily adapted to:
    a. line angles

    b. interproximal surfaces

    c. buccal and lingual surfaces

    d. calculus at the epithelial attachment

    e. none of the above

3. The primary function of the file is to:

    a. remove heavy supragingival calculus

    b. fracture heavy tenacious calculus

    c. completely remove heavy subgingival calculus

    d. root plane

4. Which of the following is *not* true of the file?

    a. it has a series of straight cutting edges

    b. its working end is an extension of the shank

    c. its cutting edges may be at 90 to 105 degrees to the base of the shank

    d. it has only one type of design for the base

5. Calculus roughened by the file should be subsequently removed with the:

    a. hoe

    b. curette

    c. straight sickle

    d. modified sickle

See Answer Key on page 227 for correct responses.

Performance Checklist for Lesson C: Removing Calculus with the File

Name _____

School _____

Date _____

	#1		#2	
	SATISFACTORY	UNSATISFACTORY	SATISFACTORY	UNSATISFACTORY
3. Demonstrate the technique for removal of gross calculus from the distal, buccal and mesial surfaces of an extracted tooth using files.				
4. Demonstrate the use of files on the four surfaces (distal, buccal, mesial and lingual) of the mandibular right firts molar of the manikin.				

Instructor _____

Performance Check Time _____

Comments: _____

_____

_____

_____

Lesson D: *Removing Calculus with Ultrasonic Scaling Devices*

A very useful adjunct to conventional hand-scaling procedures for gross calculus removal is the ultrasonic scaling device. Ultrasonic units are composed of an electric power generator, which delivers mechanical energy (in the form of high-frequency vibrations) to a handpiece into which a variety of specially designed tips may be inserted. When the unit is activated and the tip is brought into contact with calculus, this vibrational energy is transmitted to the deposit, causing it to fracture and be dislodged from the tooth surface. It should be emphasized here that the fracture will occur only if the vibrating tip is actually in contact with the deposit.

Because ultrasonic vibrations liberate a great deal of heat, the ultrasonic scaling unit has a cooling system built into it. Water is circulated through the handpiece and exists as a spray through a tube just behind the tip. This water spray also serves to flush the dislodged calculus and debris from the sulcus. Control of this water flow can quickly become a problem for both the operator and the patient. Care should be taken to adjust the water spray before beginning and to employ some means of evacuating the water from the patient's mouth as it accumulates. Either an aspirator or saliva ejector may be used, but it is important for you to be aware that these often become clogged with debris which must be cleared. It is wise to protect the patient's clothing with a plastic drape.

You can probably visualize how quickly and easily the ultrasonic instrument removes even very heavy deposits of calculus and stain. It can save you a good deal of time and energy if you are able to employ it for this type of case. It is also useful in the initial treatment of patients suffering from acute necrotizing ulcerative gingivitis. In these cases, it is thought that ultrasonic scaling involves less tissue manipulation and injury than hand scaling. This usually results in less discomfort for the patient both during and after the procedure.

Ultrasonic scaling has some limitations that are important to recognize. Ultrasonic tips and handles must be bulkier in design than the corresponding parts of curettes. It has been found that the tips must also be blunted to prevent their scratching or gouging the tooth surface and to prevent tissue trauma. Because the tip will burn both the tooth surface and the gingival tissue if it is left in contact with them too long, working strokes must be rapid and light. All of these factors contribute to the impairment of tactile sensitivity. Also, the operator's vision is hampered by the water spray.

Because of these limitations, ultrasonic scaling cannot be complete in itself. It is not suitable for definitive scaling or root planing. No matter how thoroughly you attempt to scale with the ultrasonic device, you must repeat scaling with the curette to insure complete removal of all calculus and irregular cementum.

Ultrasonic scaling devices are sometimes employed in periodontal soft tissue curettage and surgery. They may also be used efficiently to remove overhanging margins of amalgam restorations and excess cement following cementation of gold castings or orthodontic bands.

The ultrasonic handpiece is held with a modified pen grasp and the finger rests for its use are the same as those for hand instrumentation. As with hand scaling, the handle should be as close to parallel with the long axis of the tooth as possible, and the order of instrumentation should be essentially the same.

The two big differences in operating the ultrasonic device are in the use of the foot control and the nature of the strokes. The foot control must be pressed before you begin working on an area and released at short, regular intervals to allow the saliva ejector or aspirator to clear the area of excess water. Use short, vertical or oblique strokes and apply only very light pressure to the tooth. You should scale with a "feather" touch because all you need do is touch the calculus with the tip, and the ultrasonic vibrations will dislodge the deposit. Keep the tip constantly in motion. If you let the tip rest on one spot on the tooth too long, it will burn the tooth surface and the tissue; you must therefore use rapid strokes and refrain from using excessive instrumentation on an area.

Once you have dislodged a deposit, you may or may not be able to estimate just how much has been removed by relying on the blunt ultrasonic tip. It is best to stop after you have scaled several teeth or a quadrant to check subgingivally with your explorer. When you are sure that you have done a thorough gross scaling, complete the prophylaxis with your curettes or reschedule the patient for another appointment for the next week to continue scaling with hand instruments. Always remember that the last instrument you use in the mouth should be the curette.

Review Questions for Lesson D: Removing Calculus with Ultrasonic Scaling Devices

1. The ultrasonic scaler only dislodges calculus that:
    a. is already loose
    b. is in direct contact with the tip
    c. has been formed recently
    d. is located on interproximal surfaces

2. The function of the water that circulates through the handpiece and exits as a spray is:
    a. to serve as a cooling system
    b. to act as an anesthetic
    c. to lubricate the moving parts of the handpiece
    d. to clear debris from the sulcus
    e. a, c, and d
    f. a and d only

3. The ultrasonic tip should not be allowed to remain on the tooth surface too long because it will:
   a. burn the tooth surface
   b. burnish the calculus into the root
   c. lacerate the sulcular epithelium
   d. stop the vibrations in the tip

4. Which of the following features of the ultrasonic scaling device does *not* contribute directly or indirectly to the impairment of tactile sensitivity?
   a. the blunt tip
   b. bulky design
   c. vibrational energy
   d. water spray

5. After scaling with the ultrasonic scaler, when should you follow with use of the curette?
   a. rarely; it is totally unnecessary
   b. only if you do not have time to finish with the ultrasonic
   c. only when required to by your employer
   d. always, to assure complete calculus removal
   e. only upon patient request

See Answer Key on page 227 for correct responses.

Lesson E: *Use of Topical and Local Anesthetics*

When scaling is not tolerated by patients because of their tissue or tooth sensitivity, or apprehension, anesthesia is indicated. Anesthetics may be applied topically or locally (injected).

Topical anesthetics are indicated to alleviate tissue discomfort and to psychologically relieve patient anxiety. These agents act on the terminal nerve endings by absorption through the mucosa. They are short-acting and are more readily absorbed through non-keratinized or para-keratinized oral epithelium (buccal mucosa, vestibule, floor of the mouth, etc.) than through keratinized oral epithelium (gingiva, hard palate).

Many topical preparations are available. Lidocaine (Xylocaine) is the most commonly used. It can be purchased as a spray, ointment, liquid, gel, or viscous solution. Concentrations may range from approximately 18 to 2 percent.

Topical anesthetics can be applied with a cotton pellet or syringe. The tissue should first be dried with air to prevent dilution and increase absorption. Then, the anesthetic should be applied to the marginal gingiva and allowed to flow interproximally and subgingivally. Application with a large-gauge syringe may facilitate insertion into the gingival sulcus or pocket. *Absorption here is rapid because the sulcular epithelium is not keratinized.* Because of the potential toxicity of topical anesthetics, it is important to limit the amount applied, the concentration used, and the working area.

One of the disadvantages of using a topical anesthetic is that it lubricates the teeth, making it difficult to maintain a good finger rest. If you wipe the excess away with a gauze square, this problem will be alleviated.

Certain precautions should be considered in using topical anesthetics. Always take a medical history to rule out sensitivity to the drug. Tell the patient that you are using an anesthetic, and that he will experience numbness soon after it is applied. Caution him not to swallow while you are applying the topical. Keep his head in an upright position during application to avoid excess flow into the throat. If the soft palate, uvula, and throat become anesthetized, the patient may begin coughing, gagging, and complain of a "lump" in his throat or of inability to swallow. These are symptoms indicating that some of the topical has been absorbed in the throat area. Explain what has happened and reassure him that this feeling will subside momentarily. Patients often panic because they interpret these symptoms as suffocation and have difficulty breathing. A thorough explanation and reassurance should relieve the patient's anxiety.

Of all the topical anesthetics, the spray or aerosol type is the least desirable. Spray topicals are often of concentrations higher than those of the other types. It is difficult, if not impossible, to control the amount of anesthetic applied to any given area. Because you are using a compressed fluid, greater surface area is covered by the mist during application. This can become critically important if the spray is inhaled by the patient and comes into contact with the highly absorptive oral-pharyngeal mucosa. Greater uptake of the drug here can increase the chance of a toxic reaction.

Local anesthetics that are injected through infiltration or block anesthesia are reserved for extreme situations in which the tissue or teeth are highly sensitive, soft tissue curettage is to be performed, and/or patient tolerance is very low. Such cases are likely when patients are suffering from acute necrotizing ulcerative gingivitis, periodontal abscess, or hypersensitive root surfaces. MODULE V: Root Planing Procedure will provide a more detailed description of local anesthesia.

Review Questions for Lesson E: Use of Topical and Local Anesthetics

1. Which of the following is essential to insure anesthesia with a topical anesthetic?
    a. drying the tissue before application
    b. isolating the area to prevent dilution
    c. preventing frequent rinsing
    d. allowing the anesthetic to flow interproximally
    e. all of the above

2. Which of the four major types of topical anesthetics is the least desirable?
    a. gel
    b. spray
    c. ointment
    d. liquid

3. Because of the potential toxicity of topical anesthetics, it is important to limit:

    a. the amount applied
    b. the concentration used
    c. the number of patients who receive applications
    d. the working area
    e. all of the above
    f. a, b, and d

4. Which of the following is *not* descriptive of a topical anesthetic?
    a. acts on the central nervous system
    b. is short-acting
    c. acts on terminal nerve endings
    d. is absorbed readily through mucosa

5. Which precautions should be taken when using topical anesthetics?
    a. take a medical history
    b. tell the patient that he will experience numbness
    c. avoid application to the throat area
    d. advise the patient not to swallow during application
    e. a, b, and c only
    f. all of the above

Read the following phrases before answering the next two questions.
    1. extremely anxious patient
    2. patient experiencing extreme sensitivity
    3. patient with extremely inflamed gingivae
    4. incomplete anesthesia required
    5. complete anesthesia required
    6. patient requires soft tissue curettage

6. Which of the above are indications for the use of a topical anesthetic?
    a. 1, 4, 6
    b. 2, 3, 6
    c. 1, 4
    d. 2, 5
    e. 3, 4

7. Which of the above are indications for the use of local anesthesia?
    a. 2, 3, 5, 6
    b. 1, 4, 6
    c. 2, 3, 4, 6
    d. 2, 4, 6
    e. 1, 3, 5, 6

See Answer Key on page 227 for correct responses.

Lesson F: *Postoperative Instructions*

Following manipulation of the periodontal tissues, patients may experience some discomfort, especially when heavy calculus has been removed. This discomfort is temporary and usually subsides by the next day. It may be followed by some minimal soreness, which will disappear after a few more days.

Regardless of the degree of scaling, a rigid plaque control regime, including a vibratory brushing technique supplemented by flossing—or by some other means of interproximal plaque removal—is the most essential factor in promoting healing. The importance of proper cleansing should be emphasized to the postoperative patient. When the patient has undergone heavy scaling, he should be advised to brush gently for a day or two. Instruct him to gradually increase the pressure exerted for brushing and massaging each day, until the fifth day when normal techniques can be resumed.

Cleansing of the oral cavity by frequent rinsing is encouraged to keep areas free of debris and necrotic tissue. Any mouthwash can serve this purpose because it is the physical flushing that debrides the gingival area. Oxygenating solutions are also often recommended for this purpose. The effervescent action of these solutions provides rapid debridement, and also increases absorption of oxygen into the viable tissues. There is some evidence that oxygenating agents may cause new granulating tissue to decompose; consequently, the use of these agents should be discouraged following surgery. Because of its easy availability, the most common rinse prescribed for patients is the hypotonic saline solution (½ tsp of salt to 8 oz of warm water). There is some evidence that this solution acts biochemically to reduce edema. Also, the warmth of the water increases circulation in the periodontal tissues and this enhances the healing process.

Instructions for use of the denticator (rubber tip) are recommended for patients who have edematous, boggy, and displaceable tissue to increase circulation, which will promote tissue response. However, use of the denticator should be avoided for the first two days after scaling. Massaging should begin on about the third day. The purpose of the denticator is not only gingival stimulation; when correctly used, it can also guide proper regrowth of gingival tissue in poorly contoured interproximal areas. It is important to note that incorrect use may be detrimental and can lead to blunting of the interproximal papillae.

In rare instances postoperative analgesic drugs will have to be prescribed by your dentist. This need may arise when scaling is employed to treat an abscess or after extensive root planing has been performed.

Review Questions for Lesson F: Postoperative Instructions

1. The most important factor in promoting postoperative healing is:
    a. salt-water rinses
    b. rigid plaque control
    c. gingival massage
    d. flossing
2. Postoperative analgesic drugs may be required following:
    a. extensive root planing
    b. initial gross scaling
    c. definitive scaling
    d. a long appointment

Performance Checklist for Lesson E: Use of Topical and Local Anesthetics
and Lesson F: Post-operative Instructions

Name _____

School _____

Date _____

	#1		#2	
	SATISFACTORY	UNSATISFACTORY	SATISFACTORY	UNSATISFACTORY
5. Describe the procedure for applying a topical anesthetic.				
6. Describe the post-operative instructions which apply specifically to a patient following scaling of heavy calculus.				

Instructor _____

Performance Check Time _____

Comments: _____

_____

_____

_____

3. A hypotonic saline solution for postoperative rinsing contains:
    a. 1 teaspoon salt to 8 oz warm water
    b. ½ teaspoon salt to 8 oz warm water
    c. ¼ teaspoon salt to 8 oz warm water
    d. ⅛ teaspoon salt to 8 oz warm water

4. Warm salt-water rinses are prescribed to:
    a. increase circulation
    b. promote healing
    c. reduce edema
    d. flush debris from the area
    e. all of the above

See Answer Key on page 227 for correct responses.

ANSWER KEY

LESSON A

1. b
2. e
3. *Appointment #*

Appointment #	Date	Procedure
#1	10-14-71	Gross scaling of maxillary right quadrant
#2	10-21-71	Gross scale mandibular right quadrant
#3	10-28-71	Gross scale maxillary left quadrant
#4	11-4-71	Gross scale mandibular left quadrant
#5	11-11-71	Full mouth fine scaling and root planing

4. d
5. b

LESSON B

1. a
2. d
3. f
4. b
5. a

LESSON C

1. e
2. c
3. b
4. d
5. b

LESSON D

1. b
2. f
3. a
4. c
5. d

LESSON E

1. e
2. b
3. f
4. a
5. f
6. c
7. a

LESSON F

1. b
2. a
3. b
4. e

READING ASSIGNMENTS FOR ENRICHMENT *

Goldman and Cohen, *Periodontal Therapy:*

pp. 391, 409 (Removing Calculus with the Hoe)
391 (Removing Calculus with the File)
pp. 396–397 (Removing Calculus with Ultrasonic Scaling Devices)
424 (Use of Topical and Local Anesthetics)

Steele, *Dimensions of Dental Hygiene:*

pp. 418–420 (Planning the Sequence of Procedures for a Series of Appointments)
189 (Removing Calculus with the Hoe)
pp. 190–191 (Removing Calculus with the File)
pp. 193–194 (Removing Calculus with Ultrasonic Scaling Devices)
204 (Use of Topical and Local Anesthetics)
205 (Postoperative Instructions)

Wilkins, *Clinical Practice of the Dental Hiygienist:*

pp. 10–11, 172–173 (Planning the Sequence of Procedures for a Series of Appointments)
pp. 182, 204–205 (Removing Calculus with the Hoe)
184 (Removing Calculus with the File)
pp. 210–212 (Removing Calculus with Ultrasonic Scaling Devices)
pp. 213–214 (Use of Topical and Local Anesthetics)
pp. 241–243 (Postoperative Instructions)

* See bibliography on page 252 for complete identification of publications listed here.

MODULE V

Root Planing Procedure

1. PREREQUISITES

Before beginning work on this module, you must have successfully completed modules I through IV of the unit: The Detection and Removal of Calculus.

2. PERFORMANCE OBJECTIVES

A. GENERAL OBJECTIVE

Given a curette, an extracted tooth with or without calculus, and a manikin, the student will be able to demonstrate the use of the curette for root planing.

B. SPECIFIC OBJECTIVES

Without the aid of source materials, the student will be able to:

1) demonstrate the use of the curette to root plane one area on the root surface of an extracted tooth until it is smooth, shiny, and glass-like.

2) demonstrate correct insertion and root planing strokes with a curette on the mandibular right first molar of the manikin.

3) describe the indications and contraindications for the use of local anesthesia in root planing.

4) describe the procedure and the agents used in desensitizing hypersensitive root surfaces.

3. DIRECTIONS FOR USE OF THE MODULE

The following materials and equipment are required for the successful completion of this module:

> a curette
> an extracted molar with very little calculus, preferably the same tooth which was used for Module IV.*
> a dental manikin.*

The manikin should be set up at your lab station and adjusted according to directions from your instructor. All other materials should be laid out on the desk next to the module.

At the end of each Skills Lesson in this module, you will answer review questions pertaining to the particular skill that had just been described. When you are able to answer all questions correctly and perform the skill, request a performance check. If your instructor is occupied and cannot check you immediately, you may go on to the next lesson while you are waiting. As you demonstrate the skills listed on the Performance Checklist, the instructor will evaluate and record your performance. If your ratings are all satisfactory, proceed to the next Skills Lesson. If any of your ratings are unsatisfactory, review the exercise(s) and request another performance check when you are ready.

---

* These items will be issued by the instructor.

4. SKILLS LESSONS

Lesson A: Root Planing with the Curette

Root planing is the process of polishing the tooth surfaces by means of instrumentation. The objective is to produce a smooth surface, free of calcareous deposits. Because of its adaptability to all surfaces and to the epithelial attachment, *the curette is the instrument of choice for this procedure.*

Root planing is not a procedure separate from scaling. It is only a more definitive, more thorough, and more delicate approach to scaling. All the principles of scaling apply directly to root planing. It differs from what we refer to as "scaling" only in the sense that the calculus to be removed is extremely fine, requiring greater tactile sensitivity, and the cementum to be removed must ultimately be "polished" through instrumentation.

In order to remove all spicules of calculus, it is necessary to remove some or all of the cementum. Knowing that the objective of scaling is to remove all soft and hard deposits from all surfaces of the teeth coronal to the epithelial attachment, you should realize that there is no clearcut line between scaling and root planing. You must become proficient at thorough subgingival scaling as a prerequisite to root planing.

Root planing is to be performed on any patient on whom inflammation is manifest due to the formation of plaque on the roughened cemental surface. This condition can exist in various degrees, ranging from marginal inflammation, at one extreme, to advanced periodontitis at the end of the spectrum. Consequently, a good review of the periodontium, periodontal pathology, and dental anatomy is strongly recommended, and especially a review of the chapters on infrabony and suprabony pockets.

Because of the mode of attachment of calculus, root planing requires the removal of some or all of the cementum. Complete removal of plaque and calculus through root planing is advantageous to the patient's health because it may increase the probability of reattachment of the epithelium, reduce inflammation by removing the irritant, discourage the formation of plaque and calculus, and facilitate home care for the patient. As a secondary result, a root-planed tooth is easier to scale and, therefore, easier to maintain in health.

Subgingival scaling is a preliminary step to root planing, and it is therefore imperative for the hygienist to become skilled at it. Scaling to the epithelial attachment is not easy because pockets are not always readily recognizable. Often a pocket is present even though the marginal tissue shows no sign of inflammation or pathology. Consequently, when you are working on a patient, do not overlook the possibility of pocket depth.

While the importance of subgingival scaling cannot be overemphasized, access to these subgingival areas is the greatest deterrent to treatment, especially where there is depth and the tissue is tight, or where bifurcations, recession, and depth are all present. Nevertheless, the success of your scaling procedures is directly proportional to your ability to cover all surfaces of the teeth as thoroughly as possible.

There is no specific curette for root planing; any curette can be used for this procedure. However, because of the complications described above, a single universal type of curette would not adapt to these problem areas. Therefore, the set of curettes that provides the greatest variety of blades and shanks is generally used for root planing. Some of the most commonly used sets are the Gracey, Goldman-Fox, and Ward curettes. It should be emphasized that these are instruments of choice only by nature of their *adaptability*.

Selection of instruments is entirely dependent on the circumstances of the case presented to you. Influencing factors are: tissue response, length of the clinical crown, sulcular or pocket depth, amount of calculus and accessibility of the areas involved. These will be discussed in connection with each of the design features of the curette. The factor of tissue response is the most important variable when there is only light calculus. This subject will be covered in greater detail when blade size is discussed.

1. *Blade Angulation.*   Blade angulation refers to the relationship of the face of the blade to the shank of the instrument. Offset angulation of a curette blade allows the instrument to slip into the gingival sulcus at the proper angulation for instrumentation with little adjustment.

Although curettes have two cutting edges, some curettes that are designed for deep scaling and root planing have blades that are angled in such a way that it is possible to adapt only one of the cutting edges to the tooth. The Gracey curettes best exemplify this feature.

2. *Shank Variations.*   The shank of the instrument may vary in length and angulation. Length becomes important when there is gingival recession and/or great pocket depth. Shanks may also vary in angulation, making it possible to adapt the instrument to particular tooth surfaces.

3. *Handle Size.*   One of the hygienist's greatest problems is muscle fatigue. After struggling through several cases of heavy gross scalings during the course of the day or after a long siege of root planing, the hand muscles tend to cramp. The size of the instrument handle helps to prevent this muscle fatigue. The larger, tapered handles are ideal. The thinner the handle, the harder the hand muscles will have to work to hold the instrument, and the more difficult the heavy scalings and root planings will be to accomplish.

4. *Blade Size.* Blade size refers to the measurement of the face of the blade from cutting edge to cutting edge and the distance between the face and the back of the blade. These measurements may vary by only 0.1 mm; but this can be significant when you consider the size of the gingival sulculus. Instruments may be purchased according to the desired blade size.

Heavy	face = 1 mm	face to back = 0.65 mm
	face = 1 mm	face to back = 0.50 mm
Medium	face = 0.8 mm	face to back = 0.50 mm
Fine	face = 0.7 mm	face to back = 0.40 mm

Instrument blade size can also vary according to the sharpening techniques employed. If a blade is sharpened only on its face, the face-to-back distance will decrease, while the face measurement will only vary slightly. This method of sharpening is not recommended, primarily because it weakens the instrument. When blades are sharpened by reducing the back sides, the entire blade is reduced proportionately. Consequently, a heavy instrument can be used as a fine instrument after it has been sharpened over a period of time. Remember, however, that a good rule of thumb is not to use an instrument once its blade size has been reduced by half.

Blade size is the most critical factor to be considered in selecting instruments. Successful prophylaxis cannot be accomplished with the wrong instruments. The patient with very light calculus and tight tissue illustrates the importance of the statement. Use of a heavy instrument will accomplish only slightly more than a toothbrush would. There is no way to force a heavy instrument interproximally in this type of mouth.

The following is a list of some conditions that dictate the selection of instrument blade size.

a. *Light calculus and tight tissue:* Use a fine set of instruments. Good adaptation is important here to avoid trauma.

b. *Light calculus, with hemorrhagic and ulcerated tissue:* This condition will require a good medium set.

c. *Light calculus with hyperplastic tissue:* This type of mouth will require a fine (or slightly heavier than fine) instrument.

d. *Light calculus with thin tissue:* A prime example of this is the labial of the cuspid, where the tissue is thin over the canine eminence. Use a fine instrument here and be careful! This type of tissue is easily traumatized!

e. *Light calculus with depth and inflammation:* A heavier set is required to reach the epithelial attachment and debride the area. It is often advisable to keep a finer set of instruments close by for use as a supplement in cases where the pockets are tighter.

f. *Light calculus with heavy plaque:* The tissue response in this case may be "loose attachment" of the gingiva to the tooth. You will find a slight amount of depth throughout. Try a medium set here.

Before presenting a detailed description of the strokes that are used for root planing, it is important to understand the procedure. Learning to root plane is a time consuming job that can be accomplished only by careful practice. Do not be discouraged if your first 99 attempts are not too successful. Root planing is an art and a talent. It takes *patience* and *patients*. As in most learning experiences, your success will depend on your *attitude*. Approach this lesson with a desire to learn—a desire to become the *best* hygienist. Realizing that much of periodontal therapy rests in your hands, you sholud realize that your ability to scale thoroughly and root plane definitively is a strategic factor in the prognosis of your patients.

The novice hygienist is usually afraid to root plane. She may believe that removing cementum cannot be the answer to the problem. In this process, she is engaged not only in removing tooth structure, but also in causing sensitivity. However, it must be realized that the periodontal patient has a chronic problem. He needs all the help you can give him to alleviate and prevent pathology within the periodontal tissues. Without root planing, his home care is much more difficult because rough cemental surfaces will harbor more plaque and calculus than would a smooth surface. Also, scaling procedures will be more difficult for him and for you. Remember that not every periodontal problem can be solved with surgery; surgery should be the last resort. Periodontally involved teeth can be maintained by thorough root planing, rigidly scheduled recalls, and scrupulous home care.

By now you have developed the control and manual dexterity that root planing demands. To begin with, do not try anything you have never done. Adjust your thinking to root planing a surface rather than scaling off rough deposits.

Select an appropriate instrument or set of instruments. Consider their adaptability. Sharpen your instruments so that a feather touch will cause the cutting edge to "bite" the tooth surface—a dull instrument is a frustrating and useless tool for root planing. Next, adapt the instrument to the tooth surface. Make sure that the tooth-blade relationship is perfect. Keeping the instrument in constant contact with the tooth, apply *pressure*. Transfer the pressure from your finger rest to the tooth surface. Patients tolerate pressure exerted directly on the tooth being scaled better than they tolerate pressure exerted on the finger rest area. Pressure applied to the finger rest area radiates to the muscles of the face and jaw, causing greater patient fatigue. Begin your working stroke. You are now removing not only calculus, but also the cementum where calculus is embedded.

It is now time to work on your strokes. Every hygienist has her own way of root planing. Keep in mind that it is the end result that you are looking for—a completely smooth root surface.

The two most widely used strokes in root planing are the pull stroke and the *push-pull stroke*. The pull stroke has been adequately described in previous modules. The push-pull method utilizes a vertical stroke, which requires maximum control. To activate the push-pull stroke, you exert equal amounts of pressure in both directions to allow both the push and pull motions to be working strokes.

Initially, your strokes should be short, overlapping, and concentrated in a small area. Every stroke you have learned can be utilized to root plane; however, vertical and oblique strokes are most successful to start with. As the surface becomes smoother, your strokes should become longer and *lighter*. Circumferential strokes (which are basically horizontal) following the epithelial attachment are excellent finishing strokes. They are especially adaptable to line angles.

As stated previously, the effectiveness of root planing is dependent on thoroughness. To review: proficiency rests heavily on appropriate instrument selection, sharpness, and manipulation. Proper finger rests contribute to your efficiency. The basic approach to finger rests was presented in MODULE II. Variations on these finger rests simplify insertion, adaptation, and angulation. For example, visualize scaling the lower right first molar from the lingual. The disto-lingual line angle is easier to reach when a finger rest is established on the occlusal surfaces of the lower left bicuspid-cuspid area. As the curette proceeds to the lingual surface, the finger rest moves to the lower anterior area. When the mesial surface is scaled, the area closest to the first molar is ideal for a finger rest.

In addition to a thorough checking with the explorer, you may find it helpful to check yourself with a fine, very sharp curette. This "checking" curette is now too fine for scaling, but provides very sensitive detecting capabilities. Your finishing steps should be a thorough polishing with a mildly abrasive cleaning agent, followed by a very fine polishing agent to produce the desired glass-like finish.

Now let's take a look at each step in root planing by working on an extracted molar.

ACTIVATING BASIC ROOT PLANING STROKES ON AN EXTRACTED MOLAR

Use the extracted molar that you performed gross scaling on with the hoes and files for the following root planing exercise. You will practice the basic pull and/or push-pull root planing stroke on this extracted molar to completely smooth the root surface and remove all traces of calculus. Draw an epithelial attachment with your pencil approximately where it used to be on the extracted tooth or, if you cannot tell where it was, draw it about 4 mm from the CEJ.

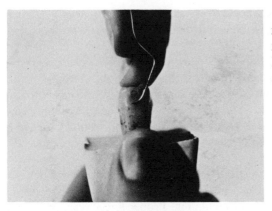

1. Hold your root planing curette with a modified pen grasp and establish a finger rest on the occlusal surface of the molar. Place the blade just above the CEJ on any surface of the tooth.

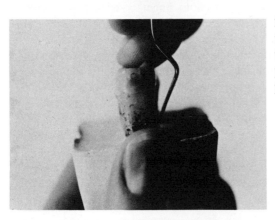

2. Insert the blade to the epithelial attachment in that area. Be sure to keep the handle of the instrument as close to parallel with the long axis of the tooth as possible.

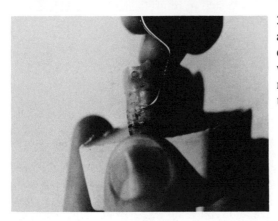

3. Apply firm pressure against the root as you activate a vertical stroke from the epithelial attachment to the CEJ. Your wrist and arm should move from left to right, pivoting on your finger rest, in order to activate this pull stroke.

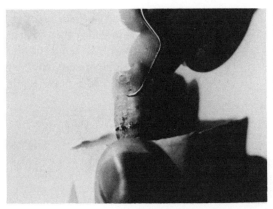

4. When you reach the CEJ, close your blade angulation slightly and prepare to activate a push stroke if you are planning to use a push-pull stroke. If you are using only pull strokes, prepare to reinsert the blade.

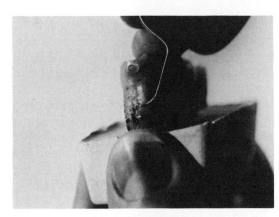

5. To activate a push stroke, return to the epithelial attachment with equal pressure. This time your wrist should rotate buccally from right to left.

If you are using pull strokes, reinsert the blade to the epithelial attachment.

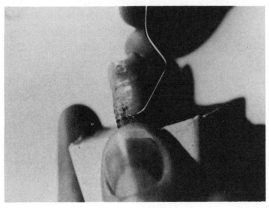

6. Continue activating vertical pull or push-pull strokes in this area until it is completely smooth and shiny.

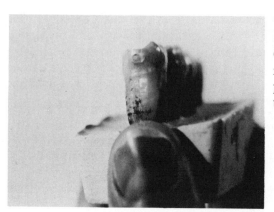

7. Examine the root surface carefully and observe the glass-like planed area. Compare it visually with an adjacent non-root-planed area, and then use your explorer to feel the difference between the two surfaces.

Continue to activate pull or push-pull strokes all the way around the tooth. When you have finished, the entire surface of the root—from the CEJ to the epithelial attachment—should be thoroughly root planed, and should look and feel glass-like.

Once you have mastered the "feel" of root planing, you are on your way. However, the next stage of development is your ability to move the instrument subgingivally without trauma, especially when working in deeper areas. Although pocket depth is not a prerequisite for root planing, you will often encounter it. Root planing these areas successfully will be the determining factor in tissue response. Reaching deep areas for root planing is more difficult than reaching these areas in gross scaling, because by this time the tissues have responded to the initial scalings. Your preliminary scaling and the patient's improved home care have allowed the periodontal fibers to redevelop as inflammation has subsided. This reaction allows the marginal tissue to become firm. Because of this tightening and decrease in inflammation, the novice hygienist is often deceived and believes that the pocket has undergone resolution. Consequently, a critical step in learning to scale or root plane definitively and thoroughly is your ability to insert the curette into these tight areas. The following exercise on the manikin will review the basic root planing strokes and also give you some helpful hints on inserting the curette into these problem areas. It is best to use older, well used manikins so that the instrument can be inserted at least 5 to 7 mm. You will be working on the mandibular right first molar of the manikin.

INSERTING FOR DEPTH AND ACTIVATING ROOT PLANING STROKES ON MANIKIN

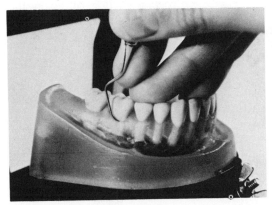

1. Establish your finger rest on the occlusal surfaces of the mandibular right bicuspids. Place the curette just above the free margin on the buccal surface and make sure the blade is flush against the tooth surface (0 degrees).

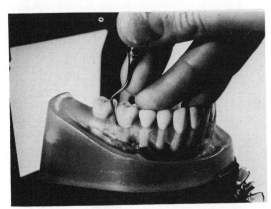

2. Slide the curette under the marginal gingiva and use the back of the blade to ease your way subgingivally. This should be a light, exploratory stroke, which is activated by lifting the wrist slightly and rocking forward on the finger rest.

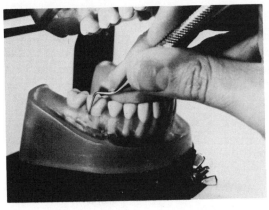

3. Once the blade is just under the free margin, make sure that it is well adapted to the tooth (especially the last few mm next to the toe). Also make sure that your angulation is at 0 degrees.

Now, lower your wrist slightly so that the toe of the curette is pointing more apically.

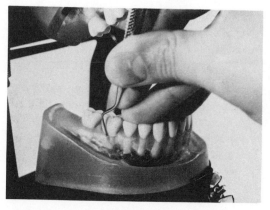

4. Then, lift your wrist and begin to gently "rock" the blade back and forth, mesially and then distally, as you slip down toward the epithelial attachment. This slight rocking motion will allow the blade to slip into the pocket even when the tissue is very tight.

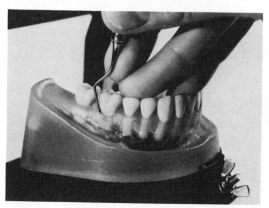

5. Continue this gentle rocking until the back of the blade is resting on the epithelial attachment. Confirm the confines of the pocket and topography of the tooth surface. Then use an exploratory stroke to come back up to the free margin of the gingiva.

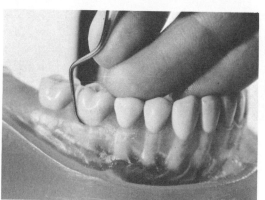

6. Reposition your blade at the free margin for insertion. Now that you are aware of the depth of the pocket and the amount of residual calculus there, begin root planing strokes.

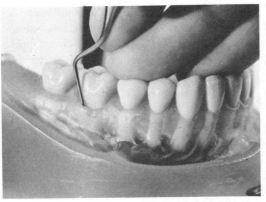

7. First, insert the instrument only a few mm and come up with a short, vertical stroke exerting pressure to remove deposits and/or rough cementum.

It is not necessary to root plane the entire root surface from the epithelial attachment to the CEJ in one stroke. Rather, it is better to activate a *series* of strokes, starting with a short stroke and making each successive overlapping stroke a mm or so longer. In this manner, a surface may be root planed systematically, with only a few long strokes at the end to completely smooth the entire surface.

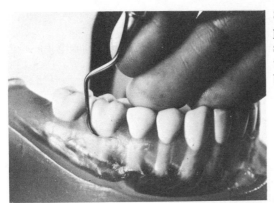

8. End your first short root planing stroke precisely at the free margin. Your blade should still be underneath the tissue so that you will not need to reinsert the blade.

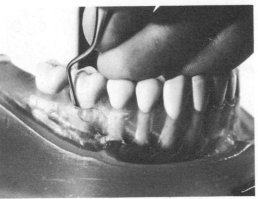

9. Insert the blade to a point just below the starting point of the last stroke. Then establish angulation and prepare to activate another root planing stroke.

If you are using a push-pull stroke, push the blade down with a firm working stroke and stop just below the starting point of the last stroke. Then prepare to activate another pull stroke.

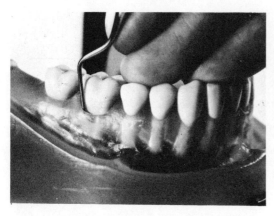

10. Activate a pull stroke and come up once again to the free margin. Continue these successively longer overlapping strokes until you have reached the epithelial attachment and are activating final, long strokes. As the cementum becomes smooth, the strokes should become longer and lighter.

The end result should be a calculus-free, glass-like cemental surface.

Review Questions for Lesson A: Root Planing with the Curette

1. What is the most important criterion for the selection of a curette for root planing?
   a. popularity
   b. manufacturer
   c. adaptability
   d. number of instruments to a set

2. Which of the following is *not* a result of root planing?
   a. reduces inflammation by removing the irritant
   b. discourages the formation of plaque and calculus
   c. facilitates patient's home care
   d. eradicates periodontal pockets

3. Which of the following conditions makes root planing most difficult?
   a. tight marginal tissue with underlying depth
   b. generalized gingival recession
   c. hemorrhagic tissue
   d. edematous tissue

4. Shank length is *not* important for access in:
   a. areas of great depth
   b. areas of gingival recession
   c. areas where the tissue is tight at the CEJ
   d. posterior areas

5. As the cementum becomes smooth, your root planing strokes should become:
   a. longer and lighter
   b. shorter
   c. firmer
   d. less deliberate

6. A good rule of thumb for selection of blade size is:
   a. always use a Boley gauge to measure the instrument
   b. never use an instrument whose blade has been reduced by half

    c. use only new instruments

    d. use only medium instruments

7. Which of the following is *not* a necessary part of root planing?

    a. good tactile sensitivity

    b. good direct vision

    c. ability to reach the epithelial attachment in deep pockets

    d. increased pressure and control

8. A thoroughly root-planed surface should be:

    a. soft and smooth

    b. smooth and glass-like

    c. hard and pitted

    d. hard and concave

Turn to Answer Key on page 227 for correct responses.

Performance Checklist for Lesson A: Root Planing with the Curette

Name _____

School _____

Date _____

	#1		#2	
	SATISFACTORY	UNSATISFACTORY	SATISFACTORY	UNSATISFACTORY
1. Demonstrate the use of the curette to root plane one area on the root surface of an extracted tooth until it is smooth, shiny and glass-like.				
2. Demonstrate correct insertion and root planing strokes with a curette on the mandibular right first molar of the manikin.				

Instructor _____

Performance Check Time _____

Comments: _____

_____

_____

_____

Lesson B: *Use of Reinforced Finger Rests*

The designs of some root planing curettes prohibit ideal tooth-blade relationships when intraoral finger rests are employed. In such cases, a reinforced extraoral finger rest will allow good angulation, while insuring better control of the instrument. A reinforced finger rest is established when a support is placed between the instrument handle and cutting edge to reinforce the blade as pressure is exerted on the cutting edge. The most common reinforced finger rest is accomplished by extending the index finger of the left hand and placing it close to or on the shank of the instrument, as shown in the photograph below.

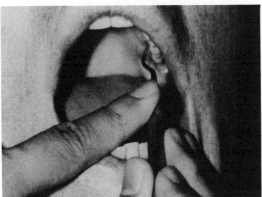

By reinforcing a finger rest, you are able to apply greater pressure to the tooth, rather than having the same pressure distributed within the instrument. Unreinforced finger rests that are established extraorally or at the end of the handle for extension are difficult to control and may exert too much pressure on the cutting edge, resulting in instrument breakage. Reinforced finger rests are most effective when working on the buccal, lingual, or mesial surfaces of the maxillary posterior teeth. You must use direct vision when using this type of finger rest because your left hand is not free to hold the mirror.

Review Questions for Lesson B: Use of Reinforced Finger Rests

1. The most common reinforced finger rest is accomplished by extending the left index finger and placing it:
    a. on the handle of the instrument
    b. on the back of the blade
    c. on your right index finger
    d. close to or on the shank

2. A reinforced finger allows you to:
    a. use an extraoral finger rest
    b. exert more pressure on the cutting edge

   c. establish good angulation on posterior teeth
   d. have better control of the instrument
   e. all of the above
   f. a, b and c only

3. This type of finger rest is most effective when you are working on the:
   a. lingual surfaces of the mandibular anteriors
   b. buccal, lingual, and mesial surfaces of maxillary posteriors
   c. buccal, lingual, and mesial surfaces of mandibular posteriors
   d. mesial and distal surfaces of the posteriors

   Turn to Answer Key on page 227 for correct responses.

Lesson C: Use of Local Anesthetics

With dental hygiene on the threshold of expanded duties, it is probable that within the near future more and more states will be allowing hygienists to administer local anesthesia. Whether or not this happens, your dentist will always be willing to give anesthesia when necessary.

Local anesthesia should be reserved for patients who have extreme hypersensitivity or are being treated for a painful periodontal abscess by scaling and curettage. Local anesthesia reduces operative time, but tends to increase anxiety in patients and can lead to greater postoperative discomfort because the patient can tolerate heavier instrumentation under anesthesia to compensate for poor technique.

Remember that once a patient is given a local anesthetic, he is generally afraid to be scaled without it. Often patients become dependent on these injections, which subsequently are not necessary.

For those patients whose sensitivity is largely a result of anxiety, apply a topical anesthetic first. Topical anesthetics are very effective psychologically. Because dental visits are stressful situations for many people, anxiety is common. Reassurance from you can help substantially to reduce a patient's anxiety and thereby help him cope with hypersensitivity. The whole area of pain is, of course, subjective and hard to define precisely. You will have to learn to recognize those instances when, despite your efforts, the patient will be unable to cope with hypersensitivity. In these cases a local anesthetic injection is indicated.

Review Questions for Lesson C: Use of Local Anesthetics

1. Local anesthesia is recommended:
   a. for all sensitive patients
   b. for patients who are very nervous
   c. when extreme hypersensitivity exists
   d. with extreme periodontal abscess pain
   e. a and b
   f. c and d

2. Which of the following is a factor that should discourage the use of local anesthetics?
   a. it increases anxiety in patients
   b. it reduces operative time
   c. it causes greater postoperative discomfort
   d. all of the above
   e. b and c only

3. Which type of anesthetic is recommended for the patient whose sensitivity is largely a result of anxiety?
   a. topical anesthetic
   b. local anesthetic
   c. general anesthetic
   d. no anesthetic

Turn to Answer Key on page 227 for correct responses.

Lesson D: *Desensitizing Hypersensitive Root Surfaces*

Hypersensitivity is the most common problem encountered by the periodontal patient. It is one of the most difficult situations to deal with for a hygienist. Only time and experience will give you the patience, understanding, and knowledge to deal with this problem. Hypersensitivity is caused by exposure of the root surfaces due to recession caused by apical migration of the epithelial attachment or surgery. The root surfaces are covered only with a thin layer of cementum, which may be missing in some areas, leaving dentin exposed. In normal teeth the dentin is quite sensitive to thermal, mechanical, and chemical stimuli.

Hypersensitivity is often manifested by patients exhibiting apprehension, anxiety, or "nerves" all of which somehow seem to set the nervous system on a hyperreactive level. Other factors that contribute to sensitivity are menopause, menses, and psychological stress.

To control hypersensitivity, keep your strokes short and concentrated. Try to keep your blade in the sulcus whenever possible. Do not use long strokes or heavy instruments. Your control of the instruments and dexterity are the most important factors to assure patient comfort.

Instruct the patient to maintain a rigid plaque control program because sensitivity is increased by the acidic toxins of plaque. Caution your patient to avoid use of highly abrasive toothpastes and prescribe a desensitizing toothpaste. If sensitivity is severe, discontinue the use of any dentifrice, since all toothpastes possess some degree of abrasiveness. Explain to the patient that the mechanical action of the brush and floss remove plaque, and that the sudsing action of the dentifrice does not.

If there is an obvious nervous problem, your dentist may wish to pre-medicate with a mild tranquilizer such as Librium. Taken ½ hour prior to scaling, it induces relaxation, increases patient tolerance, makes the patient more comfortable, and makes your work much easier.

The most important step in dealing with hypersensitivity is to prevent it from occurring. If you foresee a series of scaling and root planing appointments, begin desensitizing at the first appointment. This may seem very time consuming while you are in the process of scaling, but it is worthwhile for your patient and for you. Root planing almost always causes sensitivity, so take the precautionary measure of desensitizing early. Remember that sensitivity is a temporary problem. It will eventually go away, even if it takes a year or two.

Many desensitizing agents are available on the market today. For the best results, an agent should be relatively painless, long lasting, rapid in action, and easy to apply. It is also important that it should not irritate oral or dental tissues. Some of the drugs used in the desenitization of sensitive teeth are:

1. Fluoride
2. Zinc chloride
3. Phenol
4. Oil of cloves
5. Silver nitrate
6. Formalin
7. Potassium sodium carbonate
9. Potassium hydroxide
9. Benzyl alcohol
10. Strontium chloride

In the application of these medicaments several steps are recommended:

1. Isolate the area.
2. Use saliva ejector to keep the area dry.
3. Dry the teeth with cotton pellets. Do not use air!
4. Apply the desensitizing agent. Do not use an excessive amount. Some of these agents are toxic and should not be swallowed.
5. Burnish with a rubber cup or porte polisher.
6. Repeat treatment at least three times at separate appointments.

Of the various desensitizing agents, the topical fluoride used for caries control is the most widely used for desensitizing because of its familiarity, ease of applcation, and accessibility.

The sodium fluoride pastes (33% fluoride) are also effective agents. Best results follow burnishing with the paste. However, there is often an acute painful response to the initial application. If this problem occurs, immediately remove the paste with a gauze square, allow the patient to rinse with warm water, and then reapply the paste. Because of this common response, the paste is best received when the patient is under local anesthesia.

Strontium chloride has become one of the popular desensitizing agents because its topical application can be followed by brushing with a toothpaste containing the same chemical. Strontium chloride is probably the easiest agent to apply; it causes no pain and is very effective. In the directions for use of this agent, initial drying of the teeth with alcohol is recommended. Keep the alcohol away from the mucous membranes; it is very irritating to the tissues.

Review Questions for Lesson D: Desensitizing Hypersensitive Root Surfaces

1. Hypersensitivity is caused by:
   a. inflamed gingiva
   b. tenacious calculus
   c. exposed root surfaces
   d. poor home care

2. Which of the following modifications of technique would not help in dealing with the hypersensitive patient?
   a. short, concentrated strokes
   b. a heavy set of curettes
   c. working slowly
   d. staying subgingival whenever possible

3. Which of the following desensitizing agents is most commonly used and why?
   a. fluoride paste because it stays on the tooth better
   b. oil of cloves because it is aromatic
   c. strontium chloride because it is easy to apply
   d. topical fluoride because it is readily available

4. What should you use to dry the tooth surface when applying a desensitizing agent?
   a. air
   b. saliva ejector
   c. cotton pellets
   d. aspirator

Turn to Answer Key on page 227 for correct responses.

READING ASSIGNMENTS FOR ENRICHMENT *

Goldman and Cohen, *Periodontal Therapy:*
   pp. 411–413   (Root Planing with the Curette)
      947   (Desensitizing Hypersensitive Root Surfaces)

Steele, *Dimensions of Dental Hygiene:*
      183   (Root Planing with the Curette)
   pp. 205–207   (Desensitizing Hypersensitive Root Surfaces)

* See bibliography on page 252 for complete identification of publications listed here.

Wilkins, *Clinical Practice of the Dental Hygienist:*
      209   (Root Planing with the Curette)
  pp. 272–274   (Desensitizing Hypersensitive Root Surfaces)

BIBLIOGRAPHY

Glickman, I., *Clinical Periodontology.* 3rd ed. Philadelphia: W. B. Saunders, 1965.

Goldman, H. M., and D. W. Cohen. *Periodontal Therapy.* St. Louis: C. B. Mosby, 1968.

Steele, Pauline F. *Dimensions of Dental Hygiene.* Philadelphia: Lea & Febiger, 1966.

Wheeler, R. C. *A Textbook of Dental Anatomy and Physiology.* 4th ed. Philadelphia: W. B. Saunders, 1965.

Wilkins, E. M. *Clinical Practice of the Dental Hygienist.* 3rd ed. Philadelphia: Lea & Febiger, 1971.